The Pandemic Pivot

THE PANDEMIC PIVOT

PIVOT

JOHN FEFFER

A REPORT FROM THE INSTITUTE
FOR POLICY STUDIES, THE TRANSNATIONAL
INSTITUTE, and FOCUS ON THE
GLOBAL SOUTH

SEVEN STORIES PRESS
NEW YORK · OAKLAND · LONDON

Seven Stories Press
140 Watts Street
New York, NY 10013
sevenstories.com

College professors and high school and middle school teachers may order free examination copies of Seven Stories Press books. To order, visit www.sevenstories.com, or fax request on school letterhead to (212) 226-1411.

ISBN 978-1-64421-092-5 (hardcover)
ISBN 978-1-64421-093-2 (paperback)
ISBN 978-1-64421-094-9 (ebook)

Printed in the United States of America

9 8 7 6 5 4 3 2 1

To all those who have already pivoted
to defeat the pandemic.

CONTENTS

INTRODUCTION

You suffer a heart attack that nearly kills you.

You remember what happened: the pain, the realization, the regret. All the mistakes that you made in your life. All the things you should have done. You never exercised. You ate all the wrong foods and way too much of them. Your lifestyle was high-stress and high-maintenance. In the face of the warning signs—fatigue, shortness of breath—you repeatedly vowed to change your ways. Somehow, in the barrage of daily life, you always forgot your resolve.

"Just give me one more chance," you plead as the pain radiates out from your chest. "I'll take better care of my health. I'll make amends. I'll stop focusing so much on making money and try to do something good for the world."

And then everything fades to black.

The next day, you open your eyes to discover you're lying in a hospital bed, surrounded by your loved ones. You're still breathing, your damaged heart still pumping. You've been given another chance.

But this time will you actually turn your pledges into action?

COVID-19 is a near-death experience for the human race. We know that we've made bad choices: clearcutting the Amazon, pouring money into the military, ignoring the poor and the marginalized. We've received plenty of warning signs, from financial crises to excessive heat waves. We either paid little heed to these warning signs or applied quick and woefully insufficient fixes. And now comes something new and different: a global code red.

The pandemic that spread throughout the world in 2020 quickly made its mark. By autumn 2020, the death toll was approaching a million, with many millions more sick and a global economy in free fall.

It also quickly became clear that the pandemic could have been worse. It could have had a higher mortality rate. It could have spread more quickly and with more devastating impact. Other pandemics have been more virulent. In the fourteenth century, the Black Death killed as many as 50 million people in Europe, 60 percent of the continent's population at that time.[1] The flu epidemic that broke out in 1918 infected as much as one-third of the world's population.[2] In comparison, COVID-19 is several notches below apocalyptic.

Just as individuals often react to near-death experiences by transforming their lives, the current crisis should force a reevaluation of the status quo. Before the pandemic hit, the planet was heading toward omnicide. Climate change, nuclear proliferation, superpower confrontation, economic polarization: choose your global catastrophe.

With COVID-19, humanity has been given a second chance. We don't have to keep trying to muddle through by following the same policies that got us into this mess in the first place, doing the same things over and over again, expecting different results. We can go in a different direction. We can learn from this pandemic in order to pivot toward a more sustainable, more peaceful, and more equitable future.

Anything less will result in little more than a temporary stay of execution.

The Pandemic's Impact

How someone responds to a personal crisis reveals much about that person's character. The same can be said of nations in times of crisis.

When COVID-19 began to spread in 2020 from its epicenter in the Chinese city of Wuhan, countries responded in vastly different ways to the crisis. China treated the virus as if it were an outbreak of political dissent, first attempting to cover it up and then using the full powers of a centralized state to contain and suppress the problem.[3] South Korea brought to bear all the managerial and technological expertise of its advanced democracy to halt the spread of the disease without fully locking down the society. The US government failed to act promptly, competently, or in a coordinated manner—while the populace showed varying degrees of compliance with an uneven set of restrictions— and, exactly as predicted by most health experts, the country was soon overwhelmed by infections and hospitalizations.[4]

Diversity can be a beautiful thing. But not when it comes to battling a pandemic. Some countries—Taiwan, Vietnam, Thailand, New Zealand, Uruguay, Slovakia—swiftly managed to contain the outbreak with relatively few casualties.

But other countries bungled the response, leading to high death tolls. Presided over by a president who initially denied that the crisis was even a crisis, the United States would eventually, by April 11, lead the world in COVID-19 infections and deaths. Following right behind, Brazil, India, and Russia have also compiled poor records in dealing with the disease. These four countries, which together represent over half the world's infections and nearly half the deaths, are all led by right-wing nationalists.

The political character of these four governments is not incidental, for all four have opposed the guidance and oversight of the international community. Along with Viktor Orbán of Hungary, Rodrigo Duterte of the Philippines, Recep Tayyip Erdoğan of Turkey, and others, the leaders of the four hardest-hit countries have worked to erode the global norms and institutions that are necessary for any united response to an international crisis. If there had been more concerted international coordination from the beginning of the COVID-19 outbreak, there might not have been such wildly divergent outcomes around the world.

The vast differences in outcomes among countries are matched by how the virus has affected people within countries. "We are not all in this together," observes Diana Ohlbaum of the Friends Committee on National Legislation. "COVID affected different countries and regions in different ways and to different degrees. Poor people and countries suffer the most and will continue to suffer for a long time. Rich countries are very inward focused, paying very little attention to the impact on other countries."

The catastrophic failure of most right-wing nationalist governments to deal adequately with the coronavirus is yet another indication of their moral and managerial bankruptcy. But it is also an indictment of the neoliberal status quo to which these nationalists presented themselves as an alternative.

The pre-pandemic world was not, after all, a prelapsarian paradise. Economic globalization, the centerpiece of neoliberalism, failed to deliver for hundreds of millions of people. The major political parties that supported this economic project lost credibility among all these "losers of globalization," which provided an electoral opportunity for the far right. Despite making some voluntary pledges at the Paris climate talks, most countries were not doing nearly enough to shrink their carbon footprints to forestall a terrifying warming of the planet. Given that the neoliberal status quo failed to treat climate change as the emergency that it is, criticism of right-wing authoritarians for their bungled COVID responses misses an important point. The under-resourcing of medical systems, the fragility of global supply chains, the vulnerability of the poor and marginalized: the pandemic exposed conditions that predated the rise of right-wing nationalists like Donald Trump.

"This pandemic has starkly revealed the flaws in the neoliberal status quo globally, which creates opportunities to build progressive alternatives," points out Tobita Chow of Justice Is Global. "But the rise of nationalism is a threat to that because it threatens to close down the space that exists for progressive internationalism."

The pandemic was a political stress test. Both neoliberalism and right-wing nationalism are failing the test. It's time to try something different.

What Has (and Has Not) Changed

The survivor of a heart attack, out of the hospital and back at home, often starts off on the right foot with a new exercise regime, a heart-healthy diet, and a stress-reduction program.

So it has been with the initial responses to the pandemic around the world.

On March 23, UN Secretary-General António Guterres called on all countries to observe a global ceasefire to focus attention and resources on beating back the coronavirus. "The fury of the virus illustrates the folly of war," he concluded.[5] It was an eminently sensible proposal. Ditto the campaign for a "people's vaccine" against COVID-19 launched by the UN and Oxfam.[6]

As many countries prepared large-scale stimulus packages to save workers and workplaces affected by the economic shutdowns, the pandemic prompted a major shift toward acknowledging the positive role that government can play in economic renewal. After arguing for years that money was too tight to address major issues like climate change, governments suddenly pulled together trillions of dollars to rescue cratering economies. Some countries, like Russia and South Korea, even announced that they would redirect funds from the military to pandemic relief. Meanwhile, the drop in economic activity—including a significant decrease of airplanes in the sky and cars on the ground—was a boon to the planet: in April and May, daily carbon emissions dropped by 17 percent globally.[7]

Portugal announced that it would extend citizenship rights to migrants and asylum seekers so that they could access health care. South Korea held an election that turned out more voters than any time since 1992, which gave the ruling party a parliamentary majority for a platform that included a Green New Deal.

And throughout the world, protesters took to the streets to demonstrate against authoritarianism, militarism, and especially police violence in the wake of the killing of George Floyd in Minneapolis on May 25.

This is a good start. But it's not the whole picture.

It is like our heart attack survivor taking a walk on the first day of the month, eating a vegetable stir-fry at some point in the middle of the month, and pausing at work for a meditation break on the last day of the month. Keep to an inconstant regime like that and another, possibly fatal, heart attack looms.

The new pandemic regime that the world flirted with in the spring and summer of 2020 was nowhere near an actual pivot. The global ceasefire didn't hold, and the people's vaccine has yet to materialize. The stimulus packages proved to be short-term fixes and mostly rescued the old economy rather than prepared for a new one, most countries plowed ahead with military budget increases, and the overall concentration of carbon dioxide in the atmosphere kept rising. Authoritarian leaders took advantage of the crisis to consolidate their hold on power, and both armies and police forces have continued to act with impunity, for instance killing several unarmed people of color in the United States in the wake of George Floyd's murder. Migrants and refugees, meanwhile, have suffered disproportionately at the hands of the state and as a result of COVID-19. The Global South—the economically disadvantaged areas of the world on both sides of the equator—has received the brunt of the pandemic.

This failure to pivot has been most palpable in the United

States, where the Trump administration used the coronavirus crisis as an opportunity to expand executive power, roll back environmental regulations, and crack down on asylum seekers, immigrants, and the undocumented.[8] But in many ways, Trumpism is just an industrial-strength version of the failed policies of the previous status quo.

"The pandemic revealed to the American public that we are grossly misspending our national resources on things that don't keep us safe," observes Kate Kizer of Win Without War. "Many folks who don't ordinarily track these things are waking up to the fact that we're spending nearly a trillion dollars at the Pentagon and yet we can't defend people from a disease because our health care system is in shambles."

It's not too late for communities, countries, and the world as a whole to change course. The pandemic will remain with us for some time yet, and larger threats like climate change are racing toward the point of no return. Even failed initiatives like the global ceasefire provide critical information about what does and doesn't work.

It's not easy to get an individual to change behavior. It's that much more challenging to shift an entire society, not to mention the whole planet. But a great shock to the system—a heart attack, a pandemic—can serve as the irresistible force that causes an object on an otherwise straight trajectory to shift its course.

This Book

In June and July 2020, the Institute for Policy Studies invited sixty-eight of the world's leading thinkers and activists to participate in eight in-depth discussions on Zoom. Their task: to assess the implications of COVID-19 for key global issues as well as the potential for transformative change coming out of this crisis. They discussed a Green recovery, the global economy, coronavirus authoritarianism, migrants and refugees, budget priorities, the global ceasefire, international civil society, and multilateral cooperation.

Those discussions now form the eight chapters in this book, which are enlivened by quotes from the participants. At the end of each chapter is more detailed information about the discussants. Their participation in this project does not indicate agreement with or endorsement of the opinions of others, including the author of this book. Their institutional affiliations are indicated for identification purposes only.

This book reflects the moment of its creation. After the first wave of the pandemic, countries are still addressing the multiple political, economic, and medical consequences. In the crush of the crisis, governments responded more reactively than creatively. But now, with more information, we can better chart a path forward.

"As a historian, I've been watching everything unfold and wondering how to get our assessments right in real time, avoiding magnifying or trivializing what we're seeing," reflects Samuel Moyn of Yale University. "If we go back to 1918–19, twice as many people died of the flu than in World War I, yet there are almost no books on that pandemic compared to the massive attention to World War I. Maybe people missed the boat. Maybe the last big pandemic transformed everything and no one realized it. How do we get things right this time around?"

Getting things right is critical, but so is doing things right.

Our heart attack survivor can understand everything that went wrong with the precision of a cardiologist. But if the survivor doesn't act on this knowledge, the diagnosis is useless and the prognosis is dire.

Fortunately, many people are in the streets, lobbying in the halls of power, and organizing in new ways online. When corrupt governments like the one in Mali fall and previously marginalized proposals to defund police departments in the United States become mainstream, large-scale change seems possible. "This is the moment when we see that some of these systems that we are fighting are vulnerable," Coumba Touré of Africans Rising points out.

Few moments in human history have been truly pivotal: the industrial revolution, the abolition of slavery, the formation of the United Nations. COVID-19 itself is a harbinger, a prelude. It warns us of what will happen if countries continue to refuse to cooperate, if resources continue to be misused, if individuals and groups continue to fail to act on behalf of the common good.

It's a warning of what will happen if we fail to pivot.

This pandemic has taken its toll, in lives lost and livelihoods ruined. We know that worse scenarios await: an even deadlier pandemic, a nuclear war, rising oceans, and a killing heat. Unless the world executes a pandemic pivot, we won't be able to repair the damage that COVID-19 has wrought.

Nor will we have the strength or resilience to survive what comes next.

GREEN RECOVERY

Farmers have long practiced the tradition of fallowing: resting the land to renew the soil. The outbreak of the coronavirus led to a modern version of fallowing. Airplanes were grounded. Many factories stopped operations. Cities emptied of cars. As a large number of people stayed home, the Earth took a time-out.

In a few short months, the results were dramatic. Daily carbon emissions dropped by 17 percent globally as the economic restrictions went into effect in April and May 2020. Because of the decline in particulate matter, the particles that do the most damage to lungs and cause 7 million deaths a year, air quality improved substantially, so much so that residents of northern India could see the Himalayas for the first time in thirty years and Los Angeles's signature smog practically disappeared.[9] Wild animals, driven to the margins by human activity, started to reclaim territory, like boars entering Barcelona and goats taking over a Welsh city.[10]

A fallow year is good for the soil, but it can also lead to hunger in the belly. And so, too, with the coronavirus. The

World Bank projects a 5.2 percent contraction in global GDP for 2020.[11] With the global economy on pause, many people have lost jobs and businesses have gone bankrupt, the largest burden falling on the poorest and least resilient.

"In the Global North, there was this notion of 'nature is recovering,'" relates Asad Rehman of War on Want. "Pictures of bears and ducks and deer flooded social media, and people said that this is one of the great positive outcomes of the coronavirus pandemic. At the same time, migrants were walking thousands of kilometers to return to their homes in India, there were corpses unburied in Ecuador, there was widespread destitution in the Global South."

As the pandemic partially receded and some economies reopened, even the modest environmental gains began to slip away. In China, the first country to be hit hard by the coronavirus and also the first to restart its economy, air pollution has already returned to pre-crisis levels.[12] And despite the short-term drop in greenhouse gas emissions, the concentration of carbon dioxide in the atmosphere hit a new high in May 2020, reaching a level the Earth hasn't seen in millions of years.[13]

Since the dawn of agriculture, and despite the practice of fallowing, humans haven't really figured out how to balance economic activity and environmental protection on a large scale. With climate change threatening to inundate islands and coastal cities, this challenge has become urgent. The global response to the outbreak of the coronavirus suggests that large-scale transformation is possible. The trick, however, is to learn lessons from this crisis—about fossil fuels, the management of the commons, the nature of the global economy, the importance of good governance, and the centrality of initiatives like the Global Green New Deal—so as not to return to business as usual.

The environmental economist Herman Daly once said the world needed an optimal crisis "that's big enough to get our attention but not big enough to disable our ability to respond," observes Tom Athanasiou of EcoEquity. "I think we just got one."

Fossil Fuels

As the pandemic began to spread, fossil fuel use fell sharply. In the United States, for instance, jet fuel use dropped 54 percent, gasoline 36 percent, and coal 22 percent in April 2020 compared to the previous year.[14] Globally, the demand for oil is projected to decline by over 11 percent for 2020.[15] Already on a downward decline for a couple years, the price of oil dropped precipitously this year, even briefly dipping below zero in the United States as storage facilities ran out of room for the oil that fewer people wanted to use.[16] Oil-producing nations, after years of boosting supply, finally agreed in mid-April to cut production by 10 percent—which doesn't approach the scale of the drop in demand.[17]

The pandemic has accelerated a trend that energy analysts have long been discussing: a peak in fossil fuel demand.[18] "Along with that, a number of climate scientists say that we might be reaching peak emissions, though not the cumulative emissions in the atmosphere," notes Thea Riofrancos of Providence College.[19]

But just as economists anticipate a global economic rebound as the pandemic fades, fossil fuel use and carbon emissions might also spike. Low gas prices are already encouraging people to get back behind the wheel. "When I drive by the gas station, I see the price per gallon under two dollars a gallon, which is extraordinarily low," reports Lisi Krall of SUNY Cortland. "That offers a lot of insight into the market forces that we have to buck if we want to get off fossil fuel."

"I'm skeptical about the decline in fossil fuel consumption," counters Tom Athanasiou. "I think the default dynamic will be a brief perturbation followed by consumption returning to business as usual." After the 2008–2009 financial crisis, consumption indeed rebounded and carbon emissions registered a 5 percent global uptick.[20]

Some energy companies, already on the ropes, were hit hard by the economic effects of the pandemic. "The crisis pulled the veil back on how much debt was compounding on the balance sheet within the shale industry," reports Brett Fleishman of 350.org. "Rigs are shutting down in a string of bankruptcies this year."

The fracking industry was already in trouble before the pandemic, and so was the coal industry, at least in the United States.[21] ExxonMobil, slated to lose $70 billion in 2020, dropped off the Dow Jones in August after ninety-two years on the stock market index.[22]

But other fossil fuel companies have certainly not gone out of business because of the pandemic. "Extractive activities didn't stop for one day because of the pandemic," notes Nnimmo Bassey of the Nigerian think tank Health of Mother Earth Foundation. "These extractive activities were considered essential services. I don't see how an oil company drilling for oil in my backyard can be considered an essential service."

Not only has Big Energy not buckled, it has sought to take advantage of government stimulus packages. Companies connected to the oil industry, for instance, received nearly $2 billion in tax relief in the initial US bailout.[23] "The crisis in the oil industry has nothing to do with the coronavirus but the US government wants to bail them out because of it," points out Basav Sen of the Institute for Policy Studies.

Public pressure—anger at greedy energy companies, demand for clean energy alternatives, a desire not to return to the previous status quo—may prove pivotal in terms of future fossil fuel consumption. In the lead-up to the 2008 Olympics, the Chinese government made efforts to decrease the terrible air pollution in Beijing, only to scale back those efforts when the world's athletes went home at the end of the Games. Having gotten a taste of clean air, however, the residents of the Chinese capital pushed hard on the government to decrease air pollution.[24] The city's record has since improved considerably.[25]

The pandemic might prove to be a comparable moment, but at a global level. "People who spend months worried about their lungs are more likely to care about clean air," Asad Rehman predicts.

The pandemic has also caused a related shift in perceptions of transportation. In many cities, bicyclists and pedestrians have displaced cars, with places like Milan and Brussels aiming to make these changes permanent.[26] "People are seeing both the benefits of reduced traffic and cleaner air and realizing the need to be socially distant in public spaces," reports Basav Sen. "Sidewalks are too confined and there is all this space for cars. So, there is this push for car-free cities."

But, Asad Rehman notes, "This push for car-free cities

hasn't necessarily impacted production in the car industry."
Despite early predictions of a transformed auto sector, this
market too has begun to rebound.[27] In China, car sales were
up 2 percent in May over the same period in 2019.[28]

Walking and biking are one thing. Using public transport
is another. Ridership, down substantially because of quarantines, has been slow to recover "due to misperceptions about
mass transportation as a disease vector," observes Thea Riofrancos. "It will be hard to overcome this public perception in
the near term."

Lower levels of use have threatened the public nature
of this transport. "We are demanding the continuity of
funding—to weather the storm while ridership is low—so
that these systems don't atrophy," says Basav Sen. "At the
same time, we are talking about the risk that this reduction
in ridership becomes an opportunity, shock-therapy style, to
privatize public transit."

Global Economy

The global economy didn't just take a hit during the pandemic. Its very viability came under challenge. The closure
of factories in China disrupted global supply chains. Key
global industries, particularly in the international travel and
tourism sector, bottomed out. Commodity prices fell across
the board and not just in the energy sector.[29] Governments
closed borders, shut down international travel, and even
imposed export controls on key products.[30]

The economic downturn also adversely affected Green
technology. Orders for solar panels and wind turbines fell.[31]

The pandemic also disrupted supply chains: 70 percent of solar panels, for instance, are manufactured in China.[32] Given the overall rise in demand for clean energy alternatives, however, this drop in orders will likely be only a blip: overall solar panel installation for the United States, for instance, is projected to grow 33 percent in 2020.[33]

The scale of demand for clean energy depends in part on government action. "Global supply chains including especially supply chains for green tech like electric vehicles or solar panels are going to be increasingly politicized," observes Thea Riofrancos. "I don't think that's a bad thing. I think supply chains should be seen as political, but different forces politicize them in good and bad ways." A number of countries, including Australia and Germany, have politicized supply chains in a positive way by aggressively pushing renewables.[34]

The most obvious breakdown in global supply chains during the pandemic involved medical equipment. That, in turn, raised questions of why some governments didn't adopt industrial policies to intervene in the economy to increase production of essential goods. "In the United States, 'industrial policy' has been a dirty word," laments Ben Beachy of the Sierra Club. "The shortage of ventilators, masks, and personal protective equipment pointed to that, but it goes way beyond that sector."

Lisi Krall agrees that the pandemic has revealed the limitations of the market to respond to shocks: "Andrew Cuomo, who's not a bastion of liberalism, said exactly what the problem is. We have states bidding against other states and against the Federal Emergency Management Agency to get the kind of medical equipment they need. What sense does that make? You cannot use those kinds of market mechanisms to respond to a crisis like this."

Still, the transition to a sustainable economy, even one urged on by government, raises some sticky questions: "How can we in a sustainable way that respects workers' rights get access to the lithium and rare earth minerals that will be needed for a clean energy economy without replicating patterns of colonialism?" asks Ben Beachy.

The collapse of commodity prices will have many negative implications for the Global South. "There will be many laid-off workers and a rollback in workers' rights as a result of the growing recession," notes Asad Rehman. "But there will also be an opportunity to rethink the energy system."

Nnimmo Bassey fears that the collapse of commodity prices will force a government like Nigeria to raise revenue from other sources, such as exploiting marine resources through the "partitioning of the ocean and the dislocation of local fishing communities. The pandemic has reduced the resilience and capacities of communities." This comes on top of the IMF structural adjustment programs that weakened systems of health care, agriculture, and education throughout the Global South in the 1980s and 1990s. The result is a significant loss of life and, he notes, the revival of the "eliminationist" strain in eco-fascism that favors the "depopulation" of the Global South.[35]

Those same austerity measures generated enormous debt that constrains the capacity of governments to respond effectively to today's environmental crisis. Large-scale deficit spending in the wake of the pandemic, for instance, "is an option open to a country like the United States, but it's not an option for the Global South," Lisi Krall notes. Just repayment of external debt—which reached $55 trillion in 2018 for developing countries—absorbed an astonishing 12.4 percent of government revenue among the sixty-three most impoverished countries in 2019.[36]

Ultimately, the pandemic revealed the underlying unsustainability, inequality, and racial disparities of the global economy. "In two months of pandemic, Jeff Bezos of Amazon raked in $25 billion by himself," Ben Beachy reports.[37] "That happens to be more than one million times what an Amazon worker makes in one year. People get that we can't return to 'normal.' To use a biblical allegory, we can't put new wine into old wineskins. We can't pump new money into the old economy."

"We have learned that neoliberalism doesn't work," concludes Karin Nansen of Friends of the Earth in Uruguay. "It doesn't save lives. On the contrary, it has destroyed the planet, threatening people's health. It destroys people's livelihoods. It's weakening public services, dismantling workers' rights and exploiting women."

Governance

A robust Green recovery requires government action, but that governance must also be accountable, transparent, and equitable. That quality of governance was on display during the pandemic in places like Iceland and New Zealand.[38] Other countries were not so fortunate.

"The pandemic revealed the importance of a well-functioning government, of leadership, of having institutional structure in place that can rise to the moment," observes Lisi

Krall. "What we see here in the United States is a complete lack of leadership, a government that is highly dysfunctional." The pandemic exposed the vulnerability of democracy itself, Karin Nansen argues: "the manipulation of elections, the corporate control of the state, of data and the media, the rise of the extreme right and the military state."

In addition to pushing for a Green recovery, civil society also must advocate for greater government transparency, particularly given the coronavirus bailouts to Big Energy. "There have been big public pushes and campaigns targeting central banks and finance ministers," Brett Fleishman notes.[39] "They were there before, but now the volume is turned up because everyone is focused on these unprecedented stimulus and recovery funds from national governments and how we can close bailouts and loopholes that the fossil fuel industry is taking advantage of and help push more money to local governments and people."

Indeed, governance in many localities proved robust even if it was lacking at the national level. "People's organizing has been key to addressing the crisis," Karin Nansen reports from Uruguay. "Popular kitchens have flourished in my country. Community gardens, exchanging seeds among farmers and urban people. It's all about the solidarity among the popular classes. It reminds us of the fight against the dictatorships in Latin America, as popular classes organized in solidarity to confront that horrible repression."

The varied responses to the pandemic by national governments not only highlighted differences in governance. They also underscored the lack of global response to what are global problems, which does not bode well for addressing the even larger challenge of climate change.

"The pandemic was not the big one," Tom Athanasiou suggests. "Yet it was big enough to raise the question of emergency internationalism. The climate challenge is fundamentally one of international solidarity. The pandemic has made international solidarity real. For example, when we get a vaccine, it will be essential that we have a coordinated international campaign to demand that everyone on the planet gets the vaccine for free. And that's just a down payment on the right to health for all."

Protest and Reaction

As the pandemic spread, one response was to assert that the coronavirus was no different from a common flu outbreak. This denialism echoes a similar dismissal of climate change as nothing but a common fluctuation in temperature. In both cases, the most vocal denialists have come from the far right, like Brazilian president Jair Bolsonaro or the militia movement in the United States.[40]

"Our opponents have not gone silent at this moment," Ben Beachy observes. "They see an opportunity to put their worldview out there to gain supporters: from increased attacks on Asian Americans since the outbreak of the COVID-19 crisis to the takeovers of State Houses by armed white militiamen to Trump's labeling of antifa as a terrorist organization."

In Latin America, authoritarian leaders have used the crisis to launch "quite brutal campaigns against environmental legislation and make a new case for corporate benefits and privileges as part of their case for economic recovery," points out Karin Nansen, not to mention efforts "to delegitimize social movements such as trade unions."

The fossil fuel companies also reacted quickly to the new world that the pandemic was creating. The other side had "faster reflexes," notes Brett Fleishman. "The lobbyists were in the hallways in government very quickly, and we missed an opportunity to match their voice." At the same time, however, he points to various just recovery and people's bailout initiatives, including one with sign-ons from five hundred organizations from 350.org and a similar US initiative with endorsements from one hundred members of Congress.[41]

In the wake of the death of George Floyd, asphyxiated by a police officer who knelt on his neck in Minneapolis in May, weeks of protest spread throughout the United States and the world. "We are in the midst of a historic uprising in the United States that has been an extremely tragic catalyst," says Thea Riofrancos. "In the fall of 2019–20, prior to the coronavirus, there was a global spread of protest around the world, from Ecuador and Chile to Lebanon and Iraq. This militant protest will continue and interact with lockdown measures around the world."

"This is a once-in-a-generation opportunity for us," argues Asad Rehman. "There's the possibility of building people power around a truly transformative agenda that connects the crisis in neoliberalism to the climate to the post-coronavirus recovery, but also contextualizing this situation around race and gender. There's an opportunity to rebuild our movements around a truly transformational and international Green New Deal that, not limited to the nation-state, is more equitable, that rethinks everything from universal services and the global financial architecture to a universal income."

Tom Athanasiou, too, hopes "that people have a more visceral, emotional understanding of what global emergency mobilization would be like. We've all had the common experience of participating in an emergency global mobilization. That's huge."

The pandemic also offers a chance for environmental organizations to link with "sister movements," argues Ben Beachy. "Black people are dying of COVID-19 at alarming rates. One reason is because of the disproportionate exposure to air pollution. You can't effectively tackle the health crisis in the US without tackling air pollution and you can't tackle air pollution without addressing environmental racism, which subjected people to decades of exposure to particulate matter that is now killing people."

Turning to a Green recovery, Beachy continues, "It's possible to find a good degree of alignment across sister movements when it's about spending money. Across unions, racial justice, environmental justice, and traditional environmental movements, we have a fairly common set of demands. We have a harder time when it comes to standards and regulation."

Indeed, as Nnimmo Bassey points out, a Green recovery means different things to people in different countries. "We have common ideologies but different histories and different challenges. These are big hurdles that have to be crossed very carefully. The same way that people are disconnected from nature, we are also disconnected from ourselves. Building trust and building connections requires intense work."

The Global Green New Deal

Before the pandemic hit, environmentalists and economic justice activists joined hands to propose Green New Deals in a number of countries. In the United States, Representative Alexandria Ocasio-Cortez (D-NY) and Senator Ed Markey (D-MA) introduced a bill in 2019 describing a Green New Deal in broad strokes.[42] In Europe, most member countries of the European Union now back a call to put the Green New Deal at the heart of the economic response to the pandemic, with the European Commission's vice president pledging that every euro of recovery funding "must flow into a new economy rather than old structures."[43] In South Korea, the Green New Deal was a major element of the ruling party's platform in its 2020 election victory.[44]

The common threats of pandemic and climate change don't put everyone on the same page, despite similarly expressed sentiments. The word "stimulus," for instance, is a positive term for those looking for economic relief, but it also suggests the same kind of unrestrained economic growth that produced the climate crisis. "We have to create jobs and livelihoods for people, but at the same time we've reached the limit on our demand on the resources of the planet," Lisi Krall points out.

"We need to be aware that there will be contending approaches that use similar language," Thea Riofrancos explains. "We will have so-called Green neoliberals. There will also be Green nationalists and even more virulent forms of eco-fascism. In that context, a Left program is distinct because it's socially just, it's focused on care, it goes beyond markets, it's worker-centered, it deals with historic injustices, and it views the international terrain as one of cooperation, not competition."

The discussions around Green recovery programs provide the Left with an opportunity to "play up the dichotomy between corporations and people," Brett Fleishman notes. "That's a theme in stimulus relief fund discourse: where's the money going?"

Some of that money should go toward boosting sustainable energy, Thea Riofrancos adds: "We should put green technologies in the categories of life-saving and planet-saving technologies." Those investments, in turn, can address the enormous unemployment caused by the responses to the pandemic. "In the process of creating that clean energy infrastructure, you create jobs, which provides a solution to the unemployment crisis," Ben Beachy points out, referencing a Sierra Club report on creating nine million Green jobs every year for the next decade.[45] "You could make a down payment on tackling racial inequality by choosing to prioritize communities of color for that job creation and investments in reducing air pollution."

Investments in renewable energy are one thing. But as Basav Sen points out, they have to be accompanied by "the managed decline of the fossil fuel industry with a just transition for extraction industry workers and their families." Also, from the standpoint of global environmental justice, "it's not possible to move everyone in the Global North into green jobs," Asad Rehman argues. "We have to think about jobs in a more profound way: rethinking what work is, how many hours should people work, what's the care economy, what's a basic income, and what is access to public services."

According to the economic theory of "long cycles," new

innovations such as the steam engine, the railroad, and computers have produced sustained economic upswings. Some analysts of these Kondratieff cycles believe that health care will be the next such driver.[46] "We need a tremendous expansion of our social welfare foundations, which has to reach beyond jobs," Lisi Krall argues. "You have to have universal health care, basic income, support for people engaged in care work. A Green New Deal has to start there, or it won't get off the ground."

Another critical element of the Green New Deal is its international reach. According to Nnimmo Bassey, "There's very little talk about the Green New Deal in the Global South—not in Nigeria, not in Africa. But once the pandemic recedes, a variant of that will come to us. I am quite pessimistic because we have a lot of work to do to reach global agreement on anything, mostly because of the disruptive man in the White House. A good starting point is what we discussed in 2010: the rights of Mother Earth. If we can come to an agreement that nature has intrinsic rights, it will be easier to rediscover connections with one another and push a platform like the Green New Deal."

According to Organization for Economic Cooperation and Development (OECD) calculations, the Global South currently emits 58 percent of global carbon emissions, with China and India contributing almost 60 percent of that amount.[47] However, in cumulative historical terms, the picture is very different. The Global North is responsible for the lion's share of emissions from 1850 to 2016 (62 percent).[48] Because of this history and the wealth derived from resource extraction in the Global South, the financial burden for any Global Green New Deal should fall to the countries of the

Global North, which can also borrow money in ways poorer countries can't.

"How do we keep the global temperature increase below 1.5 degrees Celsius but from a fair share perspective?" asks Asad Rehman.[49] "You have to tackle global inequality and not retreat back to Keynesianism but also have limits on resource extraction in the Global South and understand the Global North's historic exploitation of the Global South. In other words, we have to go beyond canceling debt to reparations." At War on Want, he adds, "We kickstarted this conversation at the global level, recognizing the differences in context and language in the movements in the disparate Global South, not to mention between the Global South and the Global North."[50]

An international burden-sharing mechanism is essential to any effort to make the Green New Deal global. "The Global Green New Deal has to find its way into the center of our programs, and there is no way to do a Global Green New Deal without saving and revitalizing the Paris Agreement, and we can't do that without a fair share approach to international finance," notes Tom Athanasiou.

Before the pandemic hit, this burden-sharing conversation often ended with governments pleading lack of resources to finance such an ambitious global effort. "Rich countries talk about it but don't want to put money into climate finance," Nnimmo Bassey argues. "We spend over two trillion dollars every year on military hardware and war, but we can't raise one hundred billion dollars for climate action? This shows where our priorities are. The climate debt proposal was shot down at the UN climate change conference in Copenhagen in 2009. We need to reconfigure this demand for climate debt and not as a voluntary contribution, like in the voluntary Paris agreement."

The scale of the governmental responses to the pandemic has changed this conversation. "Six months ago, the question of how to pay for it was put to all of us advocating for a Green New Deal," Ben Beachy remembers. "Suddenly that question is not material anymore. No one asks how we're going to pay for it when we authorize trillions of dollars in government spending and ten times that amount for federal instruments extended to corporations pretty much without any strings attached. What is lacking is the political will, not cash, at least in the US context."

But countries in the Global South can also find resources in cases of emergency. "The Indian state of West Bengal and the country of Bangladesh, which has a lower per capita income than India, successfully evacuated their populations in the face of the deadly cyclone that happened there in May," Basav Sen reports. "Very clearly they have the resources to deal with that."

The pandemic has made large-scale responses not only feasible but necessary. Tom Athanasiou applies that lesson to climate financing: "Dwight Eisenhower once said, 'Whenever I run into a problem I can't solve, I always make it bigger.' I don't think the problem of international climate finance can be solved without solving redistribution of wealth within countries. You can't do one without the other."

Chapter 1: Green Recovery
Discussion Participants

TOM ATHANASIOU is the executive director of EcoEquity, an activist think tank in California devoted to promoting effective solutions for climate control. He is the author of *Divided Planet: The Ecology of Rich and Poor* and the co-author of *Dead Heat: Global Justice and Global Warming*.

NNIMMO BASSEY is a Nigerian architect, environmental activist, author, and poet, who chaired Friends of the Earth International from 2008 through 2012 and was executive director of Environmental Rights Action for two decades. He was one of *Time* magazine's Heroes of the Environment in 2009. In 2010, Nnimmo was named a Laureate of the Right Livelihood Award, and in 2012 he was awarded the Rafto Prize. He serves on the advisory board and is director of the Health of Mother Earth Foundation, an environmental think tank and advocacy organization.

BEN BEACHY is the director of A Living Economy at the Sierra Club in Washington, DC. He has worked on economic policies for over a decade in organizations fighting for workers' rights, climate justice, public health, and self-determination. In 2015 he joined the Sierra Club to help fight corporate trade deals and build power behind people-centered alternatives.

BRETT FLEISHMAN heads the finance campaign work at 350.org, based in Oakland, California.

LISI KRALL is a professor of economics at the State University of New York, Cortland. She began her academic career as a heterodox labor economist concentrating on gender issues. Her research interests include political economy, human ecology, and the evolution of economic systems. She is currently studying the agricultural revolution and its significance in human social/economic evolution. She has published widely in in diverse journals from the *Cambridge Journal of Economics* to *Behavioral and Brain Sciences*. Her book *Proving Up: Domesticating Land in U.S. History* explores the interconnections of economy, culture, and land.

KARIN NANSEN has been the chairperson of Friends of the Earth International since 2016. An environmental justice activist from Uruguay, with a diploma in family farming, Karin is committed to the promotion of food sovereignty and agroecological, diverse, and just food systems. She also campaigns against the expansion of industrial agriculture and corporate control over the food chain, while addressing the root causes of systemic crises, including climate, biodiversity, and food. Karin is a member of the National Coordination of the Native and Local Seeds Network. Working with peasants and rural women has nurtured her understanding of the importance of highlighting the role of women as political subjects in food sovereignty and as leaders in all struggles for environmental and social justice. She was a founding member of Friends of the Earth Uruguay/REDES in 1988.

ASAD REHMAN is the executive director of War on Want, based in the UK. Prior to that, he was the head of international climate at Friends of the Earth. He has over twenty-five years of experience in the non-government and charity sector. He has served on the boards of Amnesty International UK, Friends of the Earth International, Global Justice Now, and Newham Monitoring Project.

THEA RIOFRANCOS is a 2020 Andrew Carnegie Fellow and assistant professor of political science at Providence College in Rhode Island. She is the author of *Resource Radicals: From Petro-Nationalism to Post-Extractivism in Ecuador* (Duke University Press, 2020) and co-author of *A Planet to Win: Why We Need a Green New Deal* (Verso Books, 2019). She serves on the steering committee of DSA's Ecosocialist Working Group.

BASAV SEN is the Climate Justice Project director at the Institute for Policy Studies in Washington, DC, where he focuses on climate solutions at the national, state, and local levels that address racial, economic, gender, and other forms of inequality. Prior to joining IPS, Basav worked for about eleven years as a strategic corporate campaign researcher at the United Food and Commercial Workers (UFCW). He has also had experience as a campaigner on the World Bank, International Monetary Fund (IMF), and global finance and trade issues.

CHAPTER 2:
TRANSFORMING THE GLOBAL ECONOMY

The first indication that COVID-19 would adversely affect the global economy was the breakdown of supply chains in China. When the Chinese government shut down factories in early 2020 to contain the pandemic—leading to a decline in Chinese exports of 17 percent in January and February compared to the same period in 2019—companies around the world suddenly faced critical shortages of auto parts, smartphone components, pharmaceuticals, and other inputs.[51]

As the coronavirus spread, so did the economic damage. Air travel dropped off precipitously, as did container traffic at ports. States declared strict quarantines. Businesses shuttered as people stayed home. Hundreds of millions of workers were laid off. Another 1.6 billion people in the informal economy—migrant laborers, those doing gig work—were suddenly at risk of losing their income.[52]

The World Bank projects a 5.2 percent contraction in global GDP for 2020.[53] During the financial crisis in 2009, the global economy shrank by only .1 percent.[54]

The current economic downturn would have been even more severe if governments didn't step in with large stimulus programs—amounting to $6 trillion so far in the United States and $20 trillion worldwide—that provided unemployment benefits, relief for businesses, and checks for qualified citizens.[55] A number of European states avoided spikes in unemployment by stepping in to cover private-sector salaries during the lockdowns.[56]

It's a different story in the Global South, where governments have not engaged in that level of deficit spending. "Developing countries either don't have that luxury or have been psyched by the financial markets to think that they dare not," explains Jayati Ghosh of Jawaharlal Nehru University. "Pretty much across the board, developing countries are spending less today than after the 2009 financial crisis, and this is a much bigger crisis."

The pandemic not only disrupted the global economy, it challenged its very foundations. Fear of infection undermines the interactions necessary for the global circulation of goods, finance, and services. But the foundations of globalization were already fragile pre-pandemic.

"Even before the pandemic, we were seeing a lot of challenges to the global supply chains during smaller-scale crises," notes Thomas Hanna of the Democracy Collaborative. "In 2017, when Hurricane Maria hit the Caribbean, some US pharmaceutical drug supplies and other medical products such as IV bags were disrupted for a significant period of time because production primarily took place in Puerto Rico."

A more systemic challenge has been the slowdown of globalization, what the *Economist* has dubbed "slowbalization."[57]

The percentage of trade in global GDP has fallen, foreign direct investment's share of global GDP has declined, and multinational corporations are playing a less critical role in the global economy. One factor behind slowbalization has been increased automation, which has reduced demand for the cheap labor that fueled the growth of outsourcing. The pandemic will only accelerate this automation "as corporations seek to use health concerns to speed up efforts to make labor redundant," predicts Walden Bello of Focus on the Global South.

COVID-19 has already exposed a weak link in many economies: the health sector. "Some countries have robust health systems and have responded effectively," observes Jake Werner of the Global Development Policy Center, "but many don't have them in place or the existing health systems haven't responded effectively."

In aggravating economic inequality, the pandemic once again revealed deep racial and ethnic inequities. "It's been something to behold when government responses don't in any way match the realities of how most citizens live, whether we're talking about social distancing measures for people living in slums, townships, or informal settlements, or the lack of running water, or the immediate lockdown measures with no basic income in place," says Jenny Ricks of the Fight Inequality Alliance based in South Africa.

At the same time, the pandemic has provided corporations with another opportunity to sue states under the provisions of trade pacts that protect investor rights. "Law firms are expecting a boom in these types of lawsuits in which investors can sue states because of specific measures they're taking to deal with the pandemic," reports Cecilia Olivet of the Transnational Institute.

COVID-19 is attacking a global economy weakened by structural defects, altered by technological advances, and challenged by climate change. As it recedes, the pandemic will leave behind a very different economic system that powerful actors hope to return to the previous status quo and popular movements are poised to push toward radical transformation.

Global Assembly Line

The global economy is only partly globalized. Cross-border trade amounts to only 20 percent of global GDP, global value chains account for about 70 percent of that international trade, and foreign direct investment represents only 10 percent of overall investment.[58]

But the breakdown of even this circumscribed global assembly line has had an immediate impact on everyday life. The shortage of medical equipment produced in China—which is responsible for more respirators, surgical masks, and protective garments than the rest of the world combined—has thrown many countries into crisis.[59] Southeast Asia in particular, given the region's Sinocentric organization of production, suffered immediate economic damage as the pandemic disrupted Chinese manufacturing.

"COVID will likely be a turning point in how supply chains are organized," predicts Thomas Hanna. "In addition to demonstrating the inefficiencies and inadequacies of the current supply chain model, it gives a glimpse into the future impact of climate change as it increasingly disrupts trade."

By exposing the fragility of global value chains, the pandemic will likely boost the "effort to re-localize production and reconstitute local supply chains in both agriculture and industry," Walden Bello observes. "I'm not exactly sure how successful that will be because of the vested interests behind global supply chains in both agriculture and industry." Both the Trump administration in its conflict with China and the UK government in its break from the European Union have promoted reshoring, the relocation of manufacturing back home. According to the OECD, such reshoring also appears to proceed hand in hand with increased automation.[60]

"Simply reshoring production while leaving it in the hands of an oligopoly of giant corporations won't increase resilience," Thomas Hanna adds, "much less address any of the issues of inequitable distribution and access, ecological devastation, concentrated ownership, or international solidarity."

Food production in the United States illustrates the shortcomings of such corporate concentration. During the pandemic, US farmers euthanized animals because they couldn't sell them, even as supermarkets reported meat shortages.[61] High COVID-19 infection rates among slaughterhouse workers was one factor behind the breakdown in the supply chain.

But the failure also lay with those controlling the supply chains. "In the case of beef processing, four firms control eighty-five percent of production," explains Karen Hansen-Kuhn of the Institute for Agriculture and Trade Policy. "Two are American, one is Brazilian, the other Chinese. But no matter where they're from, it's the same problem: power is very concentrated within the supply chain. Farmers have few options, and the companies are trying to raise prices and get immunity from lawsuits over working conditions in plants.

And while they claim shortages, exports to China and elsewhere continue to rise."

The same holds true in other parts of the economy. "The displacement of local agriculture by supply chains has accelerated over the last few years," explains Walden Bello. "In Southeast Asia and China, fifty percent of food distribution is now by supply chains. The Asian Development Bank has been central in promoting local farmers to integrate into global and regional supply chains. Groups like La Via Campesina have said that this is the opportunity to reassert the local chains. There have been good examples of reestablishment in some countries, but many areas are not able to take advantage of the collapse of regional and global supply chains so that local farmers can step into the breach."

Globalization

Reshoring and localization are one response to the failures of supply chains and globalization more generally. But as the pandemic increases the risk of overseas investment and corporations bring their capital home, the Global South risks the loss of jobs and tax revenue.

Another option would be "a transformation of globalization in a progressive direction," Jake Werner argues, "spreading out investment more so that it is not concentrated in individual countries. There's an argument to be made to rich countries that it would be to their advantage to expand access to capital in the Global South to create more resilient supply chains. If the production system is forced to shut down in one country there would be other countries to turn to."

Increased access to capital for capital-deficit countries, for instance, could help strengthen public health systems. Meanwhile, Werner advocates "universal labor standards that lift everyone up rather than put us in competition" to help integrate the Global South into a more equitable global economy.

Others favor dispensing with globalization altogether. "A lot of the time it's not the volume of capital but the way it comes in and the kinds of relationships it creates that all massively increase domestic inequality in our countries," argues Jayati Ghosh. "You can't just make global value chains nice. They're founded on the control by multinational corporations of all aspects of production and distribution, by which they retain intellectual property rights that allow them to transfer massive amounts of value, often for no reason other than tax purposes. More access to capital that is deeply polarizing and oriented toward the fruitless extraction of nature in our countries is meaningless, as are universal labor standards when wage differentials are one to five hundred on average."

Joining the Left in critiquing globalization have been right-wing populists like Donald Trump, Viktor Orbán in Hungary, and other nationalists. Marine Le Pen, the head of the French Far Right, "abandoned some of her old anti-tax policies and began to adopt anti-globalization platforms," Walden Bello notes. "If you look at Austria and elsewhere, there's been an effort by authoritarians to create a base within the traditional working class by cherry-picking the agenda of the Left."

The anti-globalization stance of nationalist populists in the Global North has at least partly been a function of political opportunism as they distance themselves from the unpopular free-trade agenda embraced by liberals and social democrats. "The first executive order that Trump issued was to withdraw from the Trans-Pacific Partnership," Bello adds, "which was something endorsed by both Republicans and most Democrats. This is because Trump was going to strengthen his hold on the working-class base in the Rust Belt, which was responsible for his election."

Not all nationalists oppose globalization. Some nationalist regimes, Manuel Perez-Rocha of the Institute for Policy Studies points out, are "a continuation one way or another of neoliberalism," for instance in their policies of environmental deregulation. Throughout the Global South, authoritarian governments have supported neoliberal policies, beginning with Augusto Pinochet of Chile and continuing today with Colombia's Iván Duque.

In some sense, Jake Warner argues, neoliberalism is in flux. "In the United States, prominent senators like Marco Rubio (R-FL) and Tom Cotton (R-AR) are repudiating the free-market orientation of the Republican Party in the name of a state-led nationalist and militarized organization of the economy," he notes. "Neoliberalism is repudiating the foundations of neoliberalism and bringing into existence something new."

Trade and Investment

As a result of the pandemic and shortages of medical equipment, eighty countries imposed trade restrictions on personal protective equipment.[62] Other countries restricted food exports to protect local supplies. As shutdowns multiplied, global trade in goods dropped 12 percent in April 2020, the largest monthly drop in at least two decades.[63] The World Trade Organization predicts that in 2020, trade will fall somewhere between 13 percent and 32 percent.[64]

COVID-19 put a spotlight on all the flaws of the global trade and investment regime, first and foremost the dismantling of essential public services. "Years and years of liberalization have put public services into private hands," observes Cecilia Olivet. "In the pandemic, many governments had to put measures into place to ban companies from cutting off water or gas when people couldn't pay because people had to have access to these basic services during the crisis." At the same time, she continues, "some governments are putting into place compulsory licenses so that COVID vaccines should be accessible to all—because of the intellectual property rights [IPR] restrictions engrained in so many trade agreements."

These efforts by governments to protect public services and access to future vaccines put them at risk of lawsuits by corporations invoking any of the more than 2,800 bilateral investment treaties worldwide.[65] The extraction industry is leading the way in initiating disputes against states. "Arguing that mining is essential now for post–COVID-19 economic recovery, they are lobbying to expedite executive decisions to weaken already limited measures that address the social, cultural, environmental, and economic impacts of their activities on communities," reports Manuel Perez-Rocha, adding that pending mining company claims total at least $45 billion.

For all its disruptions, the pandemic has not forced a rethink on trade and investment. "Governments are not pausing to say, 'Let's hold on a second. Twenty years of this trade and investment regime has caused all of this, maybe we should change course,'" Cecilia Olivet notes. "Instead, they're saying, 'Let's do more of the same but quicker to get out of recession.' The EU, for instance, is signing new investment agreements at a faster pace."

Nor have trade talks in general hit pause. The United States and United Kingdom are moving forward with a post-Brexit trade deal, "which will lock in some of the bad deregulatory policies," reports Karen Hansen-Kuhn.[66] "The United States has started trade talks with Kenya, and there's also the EU-Mercosur agreement. They've figured out how to do these negotiations virtually."[67]

Although the pandemic has reduced interactions among countries, resolving the crisis will require cooperation. "As we think about developing and producing vaccines, there will be more of an argument for what the World Health Organization calls a 'patent pool,' the suspension of IPR to develop a vaccine," she continues.

Government Responses

Governments have varied widely in their pandemic responses, from laissez-faire denial to strict lockdowns to state-led efforts to keep economies afloat. In one common response, however, more than 135 countries imposed border restrictions.[68] "There will be even greater border controls owing to the marriage of racism, disease prevention, and high technology," Walden Bello predicts, "and this will increase difficulties for migrant workers."

In many countries, there was "a failure in political leadership and domestic governance, people closing their eyes to the disease," notes Jake Werner. "We saw that in Wuhan at first: local officials didn't want to see it because it would endanger growth and their own political position within the Chinese system. Even now we're seeing this in an absurdly inflated form in the United States and in Brazil."

Elsewhere, despite hospitals reportedly overwhelmed with patients, Tanzanian president John Magufuli urged citizens to flock to churches and mosques because "the corona disease has been eliminated thanks to God."[69] Meanwhile, Gurbanguly Berdymukhammedov of Turkmenistan forbade anyone in his country from even uttering the word "coronavirus."[70] In India, where the number of cases rapidly increased over the summer, "there's absolutely no policy for dealing with the pandemic," reports Jayati Ghosh. "The government has advanced a policy of self-reliance which means, basically, 'you're on your own, we're doing nothing for you.'"

On the other side of the spectrum, South Korea and Taiwan effectively addressed the pandemic with widespread testing, contact tracing, and selective quarantining without fully shutting down their economies. In Thailand, as Walden Bello explains, despite an incompetent military government response, "we have a very good public health system built on very successful public health campaigns on family planning and preventing HIV. The universal health system, one of the best in the world, gives 98 percent of the population access to health." As a result, Thailand kept down both the rate of infections (a little over 3,400) and the number of deaths (a little over 50). A combination of citizen participation and the initiative of public health authorities ensured nearly universal face mask use and other precautions.

Minimalists and maximalists are battling in the economic realm as well, although those favoring government action to keep the economy afloat have generally won the day, if only temporarily. In the United States, as Thomas Hanna points out, "the extent to which the Federal Reserve has intervened in the financial crisis to stop this from becoming a full-blown financial crisis is unprecedented. The fiscal policy and what the Congress has done in terms of the stimulus also far exceed what was tried ten years ago during the Great Recession."

"It's potentially exciting with things said to be completely impossible now on the table," Jenny Ricks agrees. "The flip side is that we can already see a lot of the bailouts directed at the same old neoliberal spending patterns, the corporate bailouts, the tax cuts skewed toward the elite." On the other hand, Thomas Hanna counters, "all of these interventions and subsidies to prop up the oil companies, airlines, banks, and cruise ship companies may awaken people to the reality that these mechanisms are available for other things as well."

For the most part, the interventions have been ad hoc. "This crisis should have brought about a recognition of the need for planning or at least the coordination of economy across regions and across different levels of government," Jayati Ghosh laments. "So far, we haven't seen it, though I suspect that it will become inevitable in the medium term."

The lack of coordination has been acute in the US case, as the federal government has clashed with state and local authorities over how to deal with the pandemic. "Unless the Federal Reserve does something to aid state and local governments, we're going to be seeing very hard-core austerity measures in the coming months and years," Thomas Hanna predicts. "A lot of municipalities will go bankrupt, and a lot of small- and medium-sized enterprises will go out of business."

On top of that, the economic interventions have largely ignored the environment. "The pandemic has unleashed efforts at reviving economic activity that rely on a dramatic worsening of the environment," Jayati Ghosh notes. "Governments are actually relaxing environmental regulations, going in for more carbon-intensive kinds of things. India is increasing investments in fossil fuel because of this desperation to increase economic activity at all costs, which brings climate catastrophes closer to us."

Labor and Inequality

Global human development is on course to decline in 2020 for the first time since the UN Development Program developed the concept, with the pandemic pushing as many as sixty million people into extreme poverty.[71] According to the International Labor Organization, the second quarter of 2020 witnessed a 14 percent drop in global working hours, which equals a loss of four hundred million full-time jobs.[72]

"One of the big things coming out of the crisis is the significant deterioration of the bargaining power of labor everywhere," Jayati Ghosh notes. "That will be further accelerated by massive unemployment and a massive collapse in economic activity and the lack of viability of self-employment in the developing world." Moreover, increased automation will put pressure on the labor market. "In India," she continues, "we've seen the mechanization of the harvest because the lockdown meant that farmers didn't get the labor that they usually get. We've already had increased import of Chinese machines that will enable a lot of displacement of labor."

The companies behind automation and IT more generally have prospered during the pandemic. "Big tech has emerged with tremendous power from this crisis," adds Walden Bello. And that includes companies like Amazon, whose owner Jeff Bezos made $25 billion alone between January 1 and April 15 and is on track to become the world's first trillionaire by 2026.[73]

The pandemic, in other words, has not hit rich and poor alike. In the United States, Thomas Hanna notes, "the pandemic has affected Black, Indigenous, and People of Color disproportionately than White people. If you look at economic trends going forward in the next couple of decades, this pandemic will exacerbate racial and wealth inequality."

"We've successfully taken down the notion that this pandemic is a great leveler within countries or between countries," Jenny Ricks concludes. "We cemented the narrative that COVID-19 has revealed the gross inequalities in our societies, historically and currently. The task is to go much further and use this period—when big decisions on structural issues are taking shape at the national, regional, and global levels—to fight inequality and its deep structural causes."

Social Welfare

The pandemic quickly revealed the strengths and weaknesses of social welfare systems—health insurance, unemployment benefits, food assistance—in some unexpected places. The

United States, the wealthiest country in the world in terms of overall GDP and amount of private wealth, experienced a breakdown in the hospital system in places like New York City at the height of the pandemic.[74]

"You don't have to be a rich country to have a good public health system," observes Jayati Ghosh. "Thailand, Vietnam, also Cuba have good systems. The Indian state of Kerala performed better than most European countries, despite dealing with a union government that has been violent, vicious, and denied it access to critical resources. The public health system is crucial, but it doesn't depend only on financial resources."

As critically, the pandemic demonstrated the interdependency of social welfare systems. "If the weakness of public health systems around the world, even in rich countries like the US, is not addressed," Jake Werner points out, "then once the pandemic is under control in one country, the rest of the world will threaten it from the outside, which will increase nationalism. So there has to be global attention to creating decent public health systems everywhere."

The trend, however, seems to be in the opposite direction, at least in the Global South. "You'd think the pandemic would bring out the significance of care work," observes Jayati Ghosh. "In much of the developing world, we're seeing a decline in health care investment. What is being spent on COVID is being shifted from other health care spending. We're seeing an explosion in other infectious diseases and a worsening of other diseases that require continuous care and medication, whether it's kidney disease or TB or malaria. We're seeing a decline in immunization across the developing world and a decline in reproductive health access for women."

Roughly three political factions are battling over the direction of social spending. Neoliberals are trying to minimize the bailouts and prevent any expansion of the welfare state. Progressives are pushing for a more robust government response. "And there will be the fascists who try to cherry-pick leftist measures like the welfare state but give it a racist twist by saying that only people of the right color and right culture can access those benefits," says Walden Bello.

Many of the benefits of the New Deal in the United States were similarly predicated on racial preferences—in housing, employment, and agriculture.[75] In applying lessons from that period, Karen Hansen-Kuhn points out that it's critical "to incorporate a human rights dimension into our plans."

Geopolitics

In pandemics past—influenza, SARS, MERS—the world community converged rapidly on tracking and responding to the disease. Not this time.

"Rather than coordinate a response to the disease, it's been every country for itself," observes Jake Werner. "There's been a ramping up of nationalist rhetoric, the scapegoating of other people, partly against China, but also within China directed against other countries like the United States. There has been a worrying popular expansion of support for geopolitical conflict."

The pandemic has "deepened the north-south divide," notes Walden Bello, "with greater inequality and greater marginalization of the Global South." As COVID-19 spread throughout the Global South, hitting Brazil, India, and

South Africa with particular force, the impact has been dire on economies that are already overstretched. "How will so many governments, especially in the Global South, provide all the relief needed, in terms of medicines and compensation for the massive loss of jobs because of bankruptcies, and at the same time pay their debt as well as investor-state dispute settlements?" asks Manuel Perez-Rocha.

The primary axis of conflict in geopolitics at the moment runs between Washington and Beijing. Even before the pandemic hit, the two countries experienced rising trade conflict, disagreements over intellectual property rights, and competition for resources elsewhere in the world. Walden Bello expects "greater geopolitical conflict between the United States and China. This will be most evident in trade but in other areas too like access to technology, education, and migration policy."

Jake Werner likewise anticipates that "because China and other Asian countries have dealt with the pandemic more effectively than Europe or the United States, that will likely accelerate a shift in the global economy toward Asia, which in turn will further exacerbate a deep insecurity particularly in the United States and Europe about the loss of global hegemony and economic dynamism. In the worst case, that makes it more likely that China will be emboldened to try to exclude the United States from the Asia-Pacific region and the United States will be ever more determined to remain there to take advantage of economic opportunities."

Conflict has escalated outside this axis as well, for instance between China and India or China and the countries around the South China Sea. Nationalism is on the rise not only in China but in India and a number of other countries. "We are underestimating the extent to which different regimes and authoritarian leaders will try to use these conflicts to create situations that ultimately they won't be able to control," concludes Jayati Ghosh.

Movement Responses

The obvious failures of laissez-faire economics to address the fallout from the pandemic has led to three different popular responses. Given the absence of adequate government response, the first has been direct action. "We've seen in most countries millions of people engaged in helping their families, their neighbors, their communities in immediate response to the crisis with food, safety, health care, masks, and so on," reports Jenny Ricks. "We have to see that activism as relevant to movement building because it is reaching a new section of the population."

The second category has been Keynesian deficit spending to shore up the existing system with greater government intervention to strengthen the social safety net. In this category would be efforts to improve global health care systems and mobilize resources for a "people's vaccine" against COVID-19. Another demand-side approach is to strengthen the hand of labor. "One of the key dysfunctions of the global economy is a shortfall of consumer demand," Jake Werner notes. "Increasing wages and improving working conditions is how we can change the system so that it works for us." Also in this category, he adds, would be the United States and China achieving "consensus on how to restructure the rules of the global economy."

Another such reform involves existing trade treaties. "It's time to dismantle the investor-state dispute settlement (ISDS) system, and the mining industry is a good sector to start with," argues Manuel Perez-Rocha. He points to the success of El Salvador in fighting off suits by mining companies and hopes to extend this precedent to Guatemala, Mexico, and Colombia. "The opportunity to convince governments to stop signing or ratifying any new trade and investment agreements that include ISDS and terminate existing ISDS agreements has never been bigger," he concludes.

In the third category fall more systemic changes that emphasize sustainability and changes in ownership, for instance by refocusing on local economies.[76] "Much more is going on at a city level in terms of alternatives and change than at the national level," Cecilia Olivet points out. "But unfortunately when it comes to economic governance, there are limits to what mayors and municipalities can do." Karen Hansen-Kuhn points to La Via Campesina's campaigns for food sovereignty and the re-localization of food, which don't "exclude the possibility of trade but trade is not the driving force behind food production."

The Black Lives Matter protests also point toward larger systemic change. "BLM in the US received a lot of attention, but it sparked in other countries, including the UK, the toppling of statues of slavers and a reckoning with real history that's been resisted by the right," says Jenny Ricks. "It sparked increased protests of police brutality and [of] state murders of Kenyan citizens. It's given more attention to the murders of South African citizens by army and policy during lockdown. In Mali, thousands of people are very keen to see the current government fall."

The challenge has been to translate these spontaneous protests, which arise from real grievances into "a critical mass on the ground that moves from organizational strength to organizational strength," Walden Bello says. "Why is it that the right has eaten our lunch when it comes to appropriating some of our critiques?" One reason, he suggests, has been the "ability of the right to use charismatic leadership to get people who might not agree with them nevertheless to give them the benefit of the doubt." Despite his widespread human rights violations—as many as twenty-seven thousand people killed in three years—Rodrigo Duterte retains a high level of popularity in the Philippines.[77] "We have to seriously grapple with the ability of the new right to create a cross-class appeal for that kind of politics," he points out. "We need to look into ourselves and ask where we're missing the boat when it comes to organizing."

"The consensus behind neoliberal ideas and forms of legitimation has completely broken down," Jake Werner concludes. "That opens up the possibility of the most horrifying forms of right-wing politics. But it also opens up the possibility of something more progressive and hopeful for humanity, a global system that systematically reduces poverty and inequality, and allows us to confront the climate crisis."

Chapter 2: Transforming the Global Economy Discussion Participants

WALDEN BELLO is the co-founder and current senior analyst of the Bangkok-based Focus on the Global South and an international adjunct professor of sociology at the State University of New York at Binghamton. He received the Right Livelihood Award, also known as the

Alternative Nobel Prize, in 2003, and was named Outstanding Public Scholar of the International Studies Association in 2008. His newest book is *Counterrevolution: The Global Rise of the Far Right.*

JAYATI GHOSH is professor of economics at Jawaharlal Nehru university, New Delhi, and the executive secretary of International Development Economics Associates (IDEAs). She is a regular columnist for several Indian journals and newspapers, a member of the National Knowledge Commission advising the prime minister of India, and is closely involved with a range of progressive organizations and social movements. She is co-recipient of the International Labor Organization's 2010 Decent Work Research prize.

THOMAS M. HANNA is research director at The Democracy Collaborative and co-director of the organization's Theory, Policy, and Research Division. His areas of expertise include democratic models of ownership and governance, particularly public and cooperative ownership. His recent publications include *Our Common Wealth: The Return of Public Ownership in the United States* (Manchester University Press, 2018), *The Crisis Next Time: Planning for Public Ownership as an Alternative to Corporate Bank Bailouts* (Next System Project, 2018), and, with Andrew Cumbers, *Constructing the Democratic Public Enterprise* (Democracy Collaborative, 2019). A dual citizen of the United States and the United Kingdom, he has advised the UK Labour Party on democratic public ownership and has served on the advisory board of two European Research Council–funded academic research projects: Transforming Public Policy Through Economic Democracy and Global Remunicipalization and the Post-Neoliberal Turn.

KAREN HANSEN-KUHN, based in Washington, DC, has been working on trade and economic justice since the beginning of the NAFTA debate. She has published articles on US trade and agriculture policies, the impacts of US biofuels policies on food security, and women and food crises. She started to learn about the challenges facing farmers as a Peace Corps volunteer in Paraguay, where she worked with a rural cooperative. She was the international coordinator of the Alliance for Responsible Trade (ART), a US multisectoral coalition promoting just and sustainable trade, until 2005. After that, she was policy director at the US office of ActionAid, an international development organization.

CECILIA OLIVET is a researcher with the Transnational Institute (TNI) in Amsterdam, where she coordinates the Trade and Investment Program. She specializes in the international investment regime. Over the last decade, she has analyzed the impacts of investment treaties and free trade agreements in Latin America, Asia, Africa, and Europe. She is an active member of the Seattle to Brussels (S2B) network. Between 2013 and 2015, Cecilia was a member and chair of the Presidential Commission that audited Ecuador's bilateral investment treaties. She can be reached at ceciliaolivet@tni.org and @CeOlivet.

JENNY RICKS, based in South Africa, is the global convener of the Fight Inequality Alliance, a group of human rights, women's rights, environmental, labor, faith-based, and other civil society organizations and movements.

MANUEL PEREZ-ROCHA is an associate fellow of the Institute for Policy Studies in Washington, DC, and an associate of the Transnational Institute (TNI) in Amsterdam. He is a Mexican national who has led efforts to promote just and sustainable alternative approaches to trade and investment agreements for two decades. Prior to working for IPS's Global Economy Program, he worked with the Mexican Action Network on Free Trade (RMALC) and continues to be a member of that coalition's executive committee. He also worked for the Make Trade Fair campaign of Oxfam International. Some of his latest publications include op-eds in the *Nation* and the *New York Times*.

JAKE WERNER, one of the co-founders of Justice Is Global, is a historian of modern China. He is director of policy and political research at PrestonWerner Ventures and is an incoming research fellow at the Global Development Policy Center at Boston University. His work has appeared in the *Nation*, *Foreign Policy*, and *Made in China*.

CORONAVIRUS AUTHORITARIANISM

In their response to the coronavirus epidemic, ninety countries declared states of emergency.[78] Many leaders assumed new powers to close borders, impose quarantines, and shut down economies. Autocrats, both elected and unelected, took advantage of the pandemic to consolidate their own political power by suppressing opposition and targeting independent media.

Before the pandemic hit, democracy was already at a low ebb. The Economist Intelligence Unit's Democracy Index in 2019 registered its least democratic outcome since the ranking began in 2006.[79] According to Freedom House, 2019 was the fourteenth year in a row that registered a decline in global freedom.[80] In the 2020 Rule of Law Index from the World Justice Project, more countries declined than improved for the third year in a row.[81]

Democracy has nevertheless remained popular. According to the 2020 Democracy Perception Index, 78 percent of respondents from fifty-three countries felt that democracy was important for their country.[82] However, 40 percent of those living in democracies didn't think their countries were democratic, and 43 percent of all respondents thought their governments only served the interests of a small minority of people. "So, there's still a big demand for democracy," concludes Márta Pardavi of the Hungarian Helsinki Committee, "but very little in terms of supply."

As the democratic tide has gone out, a third wave of authoritarianism has gathered force.[83] Unlike the rise of fascism in the early twentieth century or the spread of autocratic rule throughout the Global South in the 1960s and 1970s, the latest wave features a current cadre of leaders who have come to power in established democracies. Some identify as populists, others as "illiberal" democrats.

In 2020, as the pandemic struck democracies and dictatorships with equal force, states sought to enlarge their power, for instance by collaborating with corporations to deploy new technologies of surveillance, ostensibly to track the virus, but in ways that might be difficult to restrain in the future. Watchdog institutions have been one step behind in monitoring the concentration of power in fewer and fewer hands. "Like always, in an emergency, those with the most resources have ways of taking advantage," notes Jan-Werner Müller of Princeton University.

Regardless of their attempts to enlarge their power, states have confronted the virus much as an elephant stands trembling before a swarm of wasps. "At the beginning of the pandemic, all governments, no matter what theory or medical advice they were following, seemed helpless against the outbreak of a little virus," observes Wolfram Schaffar of the University of Tübingen. "At the same time that the government shows off its omnipotence, it seems powerless dealing with problems coming from nature."

The state faces other challenges. Despite quarantines and the risk of infection, protest continued during the pandemic. The largest of these confronted a particular manifestation of state power: the police. In response to the police killing of George Floyd, demonstrators decried America's history of racialized violence as well as the disproportionate impact of the virus on communities of color. Demonstrations highlighting local examples of racism and police brutality spread to over sixty countries.[84] "We have seen demonstrations happening no matter what," reports Erika Guevara Rosas of Amnesty International.

By precipitating states of emergency and strengthening state power, the coronavirus may accelerate the trend toward autocracy. Or, by sparking resistance to this coronavirus authoritarianism, the pandemic could precipitate a new era of democratic renewal. As Jordi Vaquer of the Open Society Foundation points out, "COVID-19 is a magnifying lens of what we already know" as well as, potentially, a confirmation of what we already believe.

Power Grabs

Hungarian prime minister Viktor Orbán received a lot of international attention for the power grab he executed after the virus hit. At the end of March, with the help of the supermajority his party enjoys in the Hungarian parliament, Orbán pushed through an "enabling act" that gave him nearly unlimited power to rule by decree for an unlimited time. The act provided Orbán with new tools to attack his critics. Spreading "false information" about the coronavirus, for instance, became punishable by up to five years in prison. In its 2020 report, in response to this latest display of Orbán's autocratic tendencies, Freedom House downgraded Hungary, once a poster child for liberal democracy in post-1989 Eastern Europe, to "not free."[85]

"Orbán wants to show that he is on the winning side, that he's managing the crisis well," reports Márta Pardavi. "We see in the rule by decree the securitization of the dialogue. It becomes less about health care than about a war on the pandemic where there's no time to explain or listen, just a need to act rapidly. The Orbán government argues that the emergency legislation was the only effective way to deal with the pandemic, as if all other means of engagement with the public would be completely inefficient."

The characterization of the effort to contain the pandemic as a "war" provides a rationale for the rapid marshaling of resources, the concentration of power in the executive, and even the use of the military to enforce government decisions. "The language across Asia is very militaristic, such as 'battling' the pandemic," observes Shalmali Guttal of Focus on the Global South. "'Battling' has meant the militarization of a public health emergency rather than confronting the virus and disease with the appropriate resources and strategies. In many areas, armed police and paramilitary are on the streets."

In Latin America, too, authoritarian regimes "have used pandemics as an excuse to expand their executive powers through temporary legislative measures that in some cases they're trying to make permanent," notes Erika Guevara

Rosas, with the result of "even less space for organized civil society and for independent media."

The pandemic has more clearly drawn a line between autocrats like Orbán who, as Jan-Werner Müller explains, "developed a real art of populist governance and have an understanding of how the machinery of government works," and those like Jair Bolsonaro in Brazil or Donald Trump in the United States who seek the power of governing without assuming the responsibilities of governance.

These latter leaders have "no interest in delivering services," argues Sanho Tree of the Institute for Policy Studies. "They see these power grabs as a way of enriching themselves and their cronies. Think of the coup plotters in Bolivia. They appointed themselves in charge in November 2019 just at the moment when they, like Trump, have to do all the things they were never interested in doing." The pandemic has flummoxed them because it can't be suppressed like an opposition movement. "You can't repress a virus," he continues. "There's no surrender. There's no high command of virus that says, 'Okay, we've had enough.'"

Some leaders have even used the pandemic to advance territorial claims. "In Israel, Prime Minister Benjamin Netanyahu used COVID-19 to avoid expulsion from office and to accelerate the annexation of significant parts of the Occupied Territory," notes Tarso Ramos of Political Research Associates. China, meanwhile, has tightened its administrative control over Hong Kong by implementing a new national security law in July. "Across Asia, the state and corporate capture of land, water, and other public resources and spaces at the expense of people's well-being and security is expanding," says Shalmali Guttal.

As part of their power grabs, many leaders are actively suppressing dissent under the cover of coronavirus lockdowns. Governments around the world have used "the pandemic as an excuse to crack down on the wave of anti-government protests that we've seen over the last few years," reports Erika Guevara Rosas. "If you make absurd power grabs or court rulings, people normally turn out on the streets," Sanho Tree points out. "But if you have a compliant legislature, you can criminalize this as a public health threat." Shalmali Guttal agrees: "Governments have muzzled the press so much that if journalists question what the governments are doing, they are arrested for incitement to violence and sedition."

In the Philippines, where President Rodrigo Duterte has encouraged police to shoot those violating the lockdown, the courts found Maria Ressa, the editor of the independent online news site *Rappler*, guilty of cyber-libel in June.[86] "You can now criminalize opponents who will react to outrageous acts and you don't need sedition laws," Sanho Tree says. "You can imprison your critics under the guise of promoting public health."

In some cases, these crackdowns enhanced the popularity of the leaders. Indian prime minister Narendra Modi, for instance, enjoys high approval ratings, despite his disastrous record on COVID-19 as well as his crackdown in Kashmir and efforts to suppress protests against his policies promoting Hindu nationalism.[87]

"Even in places like El Salvador, where we are documenting major human rights violations in the name of the pandemic response, we are seeing growing popular support for President Nayib Bukele," observes Erika Guevara Rosas. "This third wave of authoritarianism is accelerating because it is creating a support base across Latin America. This concentration of power gives authoritarian leaders an opportunity not just to control power through executive decision making about the pandemic but enables them to question and challenge divisions of power."

The power grabs extend to the digital realm. Before the pandemic, "there was a rapid concentration of information power in both corporate and state hands," Jordi Vaquer notes. "There seem to be signs that this acceleration will proceed." The pandemic has prompted governments to extend their control of information to the medical realm—to track the disease and ensure quarantine measures. "We don't know how this information will be used at moments of political need, like elections when governments have to ensure the privacy of this information," reports Erika Guevara Rosas.

But, Vaquer adds, there has also been pushback against the digital power grab as well as against the efforts by states to control the pandemic narrative. "Because of the nature of the pandemic, the lockdown, and the economic effects, it will not be so easy to spin the narratives," he continues. "That's one of my hopes: reality will crack some of these narratives."

As for Hungary, it ended its state of emergency in June. But the Orbán government retains many of the powers it accumulated during the pandemic, including the option to declare a "state of health emergency" whenever it wants. "It's hard to let go of these powers once they have been put in place," Márta Pardavi concludes.

The Nature of the State

Economic globalization and the expanding authority of international institutions have inevitably eroded the sovereignty of the nation-state. Anxiety over the decreased capacity of the state to control what takes place within its borders has contributed to a growing nationalist and populist backlash. The challenge to state power has come as well from within, from libertarian devotees of a minimal state whose governance has been reduced to basic military and constabulary functions.

Long before the coronavirus hit, in other words, the state suffered from a slew of pre-existing conditions. "Is it the end of the nation-state as we know it?" asks Meena Jagannath of the Movement Law Lab. "That question was relevant before the COVID crisis. But now, with governments unable to meet the demands of the people, they are questioning the utility of the state."

This challenge is acute in countries like Brazil, India, and the United States where the infection rate has been high and the state's capacity to deliver essential services has been weak. "This huge COVID magnifying lens has revealed things which break some of the implicit social contracts that these elected authoritarian governments have established," observes Jordi Vaquer. During the pandemic, people have witnessed a high mortality rate in care facilities—hospitals, retirement communities—that are supposed to be devoted to extending life. There have been critical shortages of medical goods. "Essential" workers have been the most exposed to the virus.

"Trust in government and public institutions has been a

key issue during the COVID crisis, not only in government but also in terms of the health care system," Márta Pardavi notes. "Will the system help you if you get sick? Will it cope with the demand? Even for the authoritarians who can govern and are interested in governing, this is a key issue: if the health care system can't deliver, then they won't be able to project the image of a strong and effective leader."

Where the state has failed to deliver services, other institutions have intervened. "Look at how gangs have filled in the spaces the state hasn't filled or never had an interest in filling," argues Sanho Tree. "Not to romanticize gangs—they're highly problematic—but in São Paulo, Cape Town, San Salvador, gangs have stepped in to distribute soap, masks, food, drugs. The fact that gangs can take legitimacy away from the state this easily is a really good organizing tool for movements: What's the purpose of the state if it can't even meet basic needs?"

If gangs can step into the vacuum, Shalmali Guttal points out, then civic institutions can also intervene to re-envision state-controlled utilities as public commons or to devolve energy planning, governance of land, and food sovereignty to more appropriate local levels according to the principle of subsidiarity. Even the rule of law can be situated closer to the people. "What do we do when these legal systems are failing us?" she asks. "Is it possible to develop and strengthen checks and balances with bodies other than parliaments and courts? Can we fight to have people's councils composed of human rights lawyers, activists, and local leaders?"

Some non-state actors, of course, have come to the defense of the state, such as the protestors at reopen rallies in the United States and militias sanctioned by elected authoritarian governments in India and Brazil. Such militancy "has to prepare us for unruly, chaotic scenarios," cautions Jordi Vaquer, "not just orderly transitions to more authoritarian governments." One such scenario involves even unrulier actors like the "boogaloo bois" in the United States.[88] "We also have accelerationists seeking the collapse of the current system," says Tarso Ramos. "Some militias have supported anti-racism protests because they are interested in chaos, in pushing the state toward collapse."

At the other end of the governance spectrum are the states that have effectively dealt with the crisis—Germany, Slovakia, Vietnam, Taiwan, New Zealand, Uruguay. They face a different set of questions raised by their success. "For the past year, there's been a fierce conversation whether Germany could step out of coal mining and transform into a carbon-neutral economy," reports Wolfram Schaffar. "The government kept saying it would ruin the economy to do things too rapidly. Now, suddenly, there's proof that you can even stop the entire economy if necessary and communicate that necessity."

For all states, a major challenge of the COVID crisis has been to force a change in everyday behavior. For public health measures like social distancing, mask wearing, and quarantining, the public has to comply with the state's directives or somehow ensure compliance themselves. The Chinese response to the crisis "is often described as authoritarian statism: drastic measures pushed by a strong administration," Wolfram Schaffar points out. "But it's based more on a sense of public interest than most of the other reactions we've seen." In the Czech Republic, on the other hand, a grassroots movement urged people on social media not only to wear masks but to make them.[89] Within three days, there were suddenly enough for everyone.[90] "Only after this popular movement did the authoritarian populist government take it up and make it public policy," Schaffar adds. "It's very difficult for an emancipatory movement to find a genuinely democratic way to change people's behavior, to find consensus among interests."

Compliance at the international level requires transnational cooperation, which has been sorely lacking during the pandemic. The pandemic has pitted countries against one another: to access critical resources, to prevent cross-border infections, to develop a vaccine first. "Even though we should be in an age of more international cooperation, we see international competition on the rise," Meena Jagannath laments. "The drive of states not to cooperate creates a vulnerability as well as the possibility of a different type of geopolitical order."

One such post-pandemic geopolitical order is especially unsavory. Jordi Vaquer imagines a "scenario in which we see coalitions of authoritarians coming together in more explicit ways—not just a friendship between Netanyahu and Modi and Bolsonaro but more explicit forms of authoritarian cooperation."

Elections and Populism

When the coronavirus hit, at least seventy countries postponed elections at a national or subnational level.[91] Where elections did take place, voters in large numbers often risked infection to cast their votes. The turnout in mid-April for

South Korea's parliamentary election, for instance, was the largest in nearly thirty years.[92] Voters also turned out en masse in June to make President Vladimir Putin leader for life, but amid widespread charges of fraud.[93]

At the very least, the coronavirus adds an element of potential disruption to elections, even in countries where the process has traditionally been orderly. "We're heading toward an American election that, whatever the outcome, is likely to have a very disrupted result," Jordi Vaquer predicts. "This is not new for Kenya or for many countries in the world. But to know at this point that the US election will be contested is a novelty."

Autocrats inherit their positions, seize power through coups, or stage elections to give the illusion of democratic legitimacy. The latest generation of populist autocrats—like Orbán, Duterte, or Narendra Modi in India—counts on majority support in their electoral victories to give the impression that the "people" are behind them. The skills required to win an election do not, however, automatically translate into the skills required to govern.

For leaders like Trump and Bolsonaro, the coronavirus outbreak turned a chronic governance problem into an acute crisis, exposing the fiction that they'd ever intended to govern. Instead, they'd hoped, according to Jan-Werner Müller, that "everything would be drowned out by the usual kind of culture warfare."

Such a culture war depends on the populist construction of an embattled majority against various minorities demanding their rights. "In many cases we see authoritarian movements, political parties, and individual actors relying on an increasingly exclusionary definition of who the people are" and whom democracy serves, observes Tarso Ramos. "In the United States, the paramilitarization of protest spaces with militias complements the state's militarization but also provides an opportunity for performances of the 'people' that the state will now represent. So, for instance, the militarized performance of a white nation in the reopen rallies preceded the more recent mobilizations against the policing of Black lives." This, he hastens to add, applies not to populism in general but to right-wing populism associated with the rise of a militarized and racialized nationalism.

In a time of crisis, citizens want to put their trust in government, which puts populists at a potential disadvantage. "Populists thrive on mistrust and actually activate mistrust," Jordi Vaquer points out. "Populists are not very good on essentials, and they don't tend to have a strong discourse around care. In the long run, they don't have the answers for the vulnerabilities that the coronavirus has exposed."

The pandemic has further exposed the fragility of the concept of public interest, which has been made more precarious by decades of "corporate concentration and very conservative, nationalistic political power," argues Shalmali Guttal. "In India, although our health care system has been in shambles because of neoliberal reforms and the cost of medical insurance has skyrocketed, the first line of defense and treatment for COVID-19 was not private hospitals but public hospitals and health centers. That system has now completely collapsed. It cannot take the load. And the private hospitals are now charging premium rates. So, even the middle class is saying, 'Oh, we can't afford this.'"

In the United States, the recent college cheating scandal that involved several celebrities revealed the failure of the social contract. "These were well-off people, and one wouldn't have thought that they needed such shortcuts," points out Jan-Werner Müller. "In a world that has become so stratified and governed by inequality, people realize that all of a sudden unless you're at the very top, this isn't working terribly well for you either." He continues, "Just as we have concierge medicine, as we call it in the United States, in a concierge society some can benefit from privileges that are totally unreachable to other people while those at the bottom are not in the social contract either."

During the pandemic, states pretended as though the social contract still applied to all citizens equally. "The basic idea, as we've seen in Brazil and the United States: keep the economy running and privatize the risk," Wolfram Schaffar concludes. "It's what Turkish president Recep Tayyip Erdoğan was saying at the beginning: you can quarantine if you want, no one holds you back from enjoying your quarantine. But this is sacrificing potentially a whole sector of society, namely all those who can't afford this private quarantine."

Oligarchy

The pandemic has transferred power upward into the hands of those with political, institutional, and economic power, reinforcing global inequality. "Billionaires have done fantastically well during this lockdown," Sanho Tree points out. "Jeff Bezos's wealth has skyrocketed while everyone else is going out of business."

"This is what Naomi Klein calls 'disaster capitalism'—big

corporations using the opportunity to burn the Amazon jungle at unprecedented rates, secure a larger grip on social needs, and restart the building of pipelines," explains Jordi Vaquer. Shalmali Guttal agrees: "In Asia, the corporate-state alliances are being strengthened under COVID." Throughout Latin America, Erika Guevara Rosas reports, the pandemic is "exacerbating preexisting inequalities and violence across the continent. This is how authoritarian governments are propping up large corporations and imposing legislation that infringes on human rights, justice, and the dignity of people using the excuse of the pandemic."

Because of the pandemic, Jan-Werner Müller points out, "an already existing trend toward an oligarchization of nom-inally democratic policies in some countries has gotten a lot worse. In the United States, people are vaguely aware of the amount of stuff included in the emergency legislation—for the real estate industry, the insane levels of deregulation—but they have difficulty resisting in any obvious way at the moment." On the other hand, the exaggerated redistribution of wealth and power may well be the last gasp of the old order, the end "of a cycle that began with Reagan, when deregula-tion had a real justification whether you liked it or not, and there was real normative language related to freedom. None of that is remotely plausible at the moment."

The "creative destruction" unleashed by the pandemic—the bankruptcies, foreclosures, and evictions—may yet birth this new order. "With the end of the evictions moratoria and the suspension of mortgage payments may come a collapse of the economic system," Meena Jagannath hypothesizes. "There may be a fundamental restructuring that will create opportunities for groups of people who never had access to buying land. And those could be sites for experimentation of different types of governing."

The combination of pandemic and protest "provides us with the greatest opportunity in my lifetime for serious redistribution of wealth," concludes Sanho Tree. "If you don't change the structural systems that gave us this inequality to begin with you're going to perpetuate it even more if you try to reconstruct the economy under these rules."

Protest and Organizing

The power grabs, the intensification of surveillance, the redefinition of the public interest, the strengthening of oligarchies: these trends have not been unopposed. Courageous judges and legislators have worked within the system to constrain the ambitions of autocrats. Civil society organizations like the ACLU and Amnesty International have championed the rule of law against corrupt and lawless governments.

The public, too, has found a way to push back against authoritarians, even in constrained conditions. At the beginning of the pandemic, Jordi Vaquer says, "some people were convinced that we would need to completely change the way we talk about civic mobilization and that street mobilization was no longer a tool and wouldn't be until the end of the pandemic." Then, the Black Lives Matter protests broke out in the United States and spread around the world, led by members of communities hardest hit by the pandemic.

In addition to calls to defund the police and reduce military spending, some movements have advanced economic demands. "In Brazil, a rapid coalition of civil society organizations forced a minimum income scheme that's quite generous on a basically fascist president and the most neoliberal finance minister in a region that has quite a few neoliberal ministers of finance," reports Jordi Vaquer.[94]

Resistance and reaction are now engaged in a tug-of-war. "In the United States, there's a spirit of optimism around the conversations that have been broken open by the demonstrations in the street and people's examination of systemic racism," notes Meena Jagannath. On the other hand, "we see tanks in the street, highly militarized police, protest leaders painted as terrorists. The US government is seizing upon an 'outside agitator' frame to justify FBI surveillance and the singling out of protest organizers."

In addition to organizing protests during the pandemic, civil society organizations have provided critical services. In the United Kingdom, over four thousand mutual aid organizations stepped forward to help vulnerable populations get food and medical services.[95] In Iran, social workers created an independent network to address populations like children and the homeless hit hard by the pandemic.[96]

"When governments and the health care system are not delivering, who is there to help you?" Márta Pardavi asks. "Most often some kind of civil society organization mobilizes very fast and beyond its own capacity. They're the ones that people can trust and they have the flexibility to help and provide support. But it is also not sustainable. In Hungary, many human rights organizations provide legal assistance to people who are not normally in their portfolios. What will happen once the immediate crisis is over? How will human rights organizations change and hold onto their expanded mandate?"

Another key civil society task during the outbreak, Shalmali Guttal suggests, is to "gather evidence and testimonies from those most vulnerable to the broader crisis triggered by the pandemic, those working to expose the reality of the government's pandemic narrative, and those organizing resistance and actual solidarity."

Even as public protests continue, the pandemic has altered the nature of civil society organizing, much of which has moved online to platforms like Zoom. "One thing you can't have on Zoom is anything like a spontaneous encounter or a situation in which a plurality of different people come together to work out new projects," Jan-Werner Müller points out. "Everything right now is pushing against trusting people you don't know who might be invisible carriers of a certain kind of peril."

Despite these challenges, progressives should pursue a "block-and-build" strategy, Tarso Ramos proposes, by blocking the further consolidation of autocratic power and creating space to build alternatives. "If we only block, we ignore contesting for state power at our peril because then other things become possible." Blocking the autocrats and contesting for state power, meanwhile, require resources. "So far," he continues, "there's a lack of boldness, almost a capitulation to the notion of economic precarity. How do we bring this discussion of economic reality and need for resources into a discussion of democratic possibility?"

Economic inequality sustains oligarchy and also provides an underpinning to authoritarian rule. State responses to the pandemic reinforced this inequality by distinguishing between workers who can work remotely and essential workers who are exposed to greater risk at the workplace.

"The people considered essential are also considered dispensable," Jan-Werner Müller observers. "Unless somebody stands up and fights for them or organizes them, just the moral intuition that 'I depend on these people' is not going to achieve anything. Are we going to magically see the reappearance of strong trade unions and people who are going to fight for those at the bottom?"

This is a challenge not for one state but for all states. "The way that people are challenging the legal structures in the United States and the complicity of the legal system upholding these unequal structures creates a whole language and analysis of self-determination that opens up the possibility of creating solidarity across borders," argues Meena Jagannath. "None of the problems that we're experiencing are contained within borders. How can this be an opportunity to catalyze more cross-border exchange between movements and people?"

Chapter 3: Coronavirus Authoritarianism Discussion Participants

SHALMALI GUTTAL is the executive director of Focus on the Global South in Bangkok and has worked with Focus since 1997. She has worked in India, the United States, and mainland Southeast Asia. Her academic background is in the social sciences with particular emphasis on participatory education and qualitative research. Since 1991, she has been researching and writing about economic development, trade and investment, and ecological and social justice issues in Asia—especially the Mekong region and India—with emphasis on people's and women's rights to resources.

MEENA JAGANNATH co-founded the Community Justice Project in 2015, and now works as the director of global programs at Movement

Law Lab. She is a movement lawyer with an extensive background in activism and international human rights. Prior to coming to Miami, she worked for the Bureau des Avocats Internationaux in Port-au-Prince, Haiti, where she coordinated the Rape Accountability and Prevention Project, which combined direct legal representation with advocacy and capacity building of grassroots women's groups. While using her legal skills to build the power of movements locally in South Florida, she has also brought to bear her international human rights expertise in delegations to the United Nations to elevate US-based human rights issues like police accountability and Stand Your Ground laws to the international level. Meena has published several articles in law journals and other media outlets, and has spoken in numerous academic and conference settings.

JAN-WERNER MÜLLER teaches in the politics department of Princeton University. He has been a member of the School of Historical Studies, Institute of Advanced Study, Princeton, and a visiting fellow at the Collegium Budapest Institute of Advanced Study, Collegium Helsinki, the Institute for Human Sciences in Vienna, the Remarque Institute, New York University, the Center for European Studies, Harvard, as well as the Robert Schuman Centre for Advanced Studies, European University Institute, Florence. He is the author of *Contesting Democracy* (Yale University Press, 2011), *What is Populism?* (University of Pennsylvania Press, 2016), and *Furcht und Freiheit: Für einen anderen Liberalismus* (Suhrkamp, 2019). His public affairs commentary and essays have appeared in the *London Review of Books*, the *New York Review of Books*, *Foreign Affairs*, the *Guardian*, the *New York Times*, and *Project Syndicate*.

MÁRTA PARDAVI is co-chair of the Hungarian Helsinki Committee. Márta currently serves on the board of the PILnet Hungary Foundation and the Verzio International Human Rights Documentary Film Festival. Previously she served as board member, and later vice-chair, of the European Council on Refugees and Exiles from 2003 to 2011. She has been awarded the 2018 William D. Zabel Human Rights Award from Human Rights First, the 2019 Civil Rights Defender of the Year Award, and was chosen to be a member of POLITICO 28 Class of 2019.

TARSO RAMOS is executive director of Political Research Associates

(PRA), based in Massachusetts. Under his leadership, PRA has expanded existing lines of research documenting right-wing attacks on reproductive, gender, and racial justice by launching several new initiatives on subjects that include the export of US-style homophobic campaigns abroad, the spread of Islamophobia, and the Right's investment in redefining religious liberty toward discriminatory ends. Before joining PRA, Ramos served as founding director of Western States Center's Racial Justice Program, which works to oppose racist public policy initiatives and support progressive people of color–led organizations. As director of the Wise Use Public Exposure Project in the mid-1990s, he tracked the Right's anti-union and anti-environmental campaigns. As an activist-in-residence at the Barnard Center for Research on Women, Ramos worked on addressing authoritarianism and misogyny as well as examining gender and white supremacy.

ERIKA GUEVARA ROSAS is a Mexican-American human rights lawyer and feminist activist who currently serves as the Americas director at Amnesty International, where she leads the organization's human rights work across the continent. She brings more than twenty years of experience in social and gender justice, human rights, and philanthropy.

WOLFRAM SCHAFFAR is a professor of Japanese studies at the University of Tübingen and an associated researcher in the Department of Southeast Asian Studies, University of Passau. From 2010 until 2018, he was a professor of development studies and political science in the Department of Development Studies at the University of Vienna. Prior to this, he was affiliated with the University of Bonn, Chulalongkorn University in Bangkok, and the Royal Netherlands Institute of Southeast Asian and Caribbean Studies (KITLV) in Leiden, Netherlands. His fields of interest are state theory of the Global South, social movements, new constitutionalism, and democratization processes, as well as the new authoritarianism.

SANHO TREE is a fellow at the Institute for Policy Studies in Washington, DC, and has been director of its Drug Policy Project since 1998. A former military and diplomatic historian, his current work encompasses the reform of both international and domestic drug policies by promoting alternatives to the failed prohibitionist model. He previously collaborated with Gar Alperovitz on *The Decision to Use the Atomic Bomb and the Architecture of an American Myth* (Knopf, 1995). He was also associate editor of *CovertAction Quarterly*, an award-winning magazine of investigative journalism, and he worked at the International Human Rights Law Group in the late 1980s. Currently, he serves on the board of the Andean Information Network.

JORDI VAQUER is the director for Global Foresight and Analysis at the Open Society Foundations. Previously, he was the Open Society Foundations regional director for Europe and a co-director of the Open Society Initiative for Europe. He is an affiliated lecturer at the Barcelona Institute for International Affairs and a regular contributor to Spanish media on international affairs and EU politics. Before joining the Open Society Foundations, he was director of the Barcelona Centre for International Affairs, one of southern Europe's most influential international relations think tanks.

CHAPTER 4:
RETHINKING BORDERS AND MIGRATION

The novel coronavirus has devastated many communities: the elderly, the poor, those with preexisting conditions like diabetes. But the population perhaps most adversely affected has been the migrant and refugee community.

Even before the pandemic hit, more people had been displaced by conflict—as refugees, asylum seekers, or internally displaced—than at any time since World War II.[97] By the end of 2019, nearly eighty million people were on the move because of war, violence, and persecution. Almost 70 percent of this number came from just five countries: Syria, Venezuela, Afghanistan, South Sudan, and Myanmar. Forty percent of this number are children.[98]

The pandemic didn't stop these conflicts, but it did prompt governments to shut down borders and freeze asylum processing. The UN, too, stopped all refugee resettlement.[99] "The refugee and migrant community is nervous that it won't restart again or, if it does, that it won't restart at the same level that it was previously, which was already inadequate," reports Brami Jegan of the Stop Deportations to Danger campaign. "There's going to be a huge number of people in highly dangerous situations, who are going to move to safety using unsafe pathways."

It's become more dangerous as well for those living temporarily in refugee facilities, since overcrowding increases the odds of rapid virus transmission. In one reception center in Germany, for instance, four hundred out of six hundred refugees tested positive for COVID-19.[100] At an immigrant detention center in Virginia, 75 percent of the 360 detainees contracted the disease.[101]

The border restrictions associated with COVID, meanwhile, come on top of a wave of anti-immigrant measures imposed throughout the Global North. "What we're seeing in terms of migrants and refugees is not so much a new era of repression, detention, and pushback but an intensification," observes Brid Brennan of the Transnational Institute. "The European policy on migration and asylum is really being enforced heavily under conditions of COVID. This is not new. What's new is the transparency with which it is done."

The economic consequences of the lockdowns have put additional burdens on a community that was already struggling to access medical care. Of European countries during the pandemic, only Portugal extended national health care to immigrants and asylum seekers with pending citizenship cases.[102] Prior to the pandemic, the only country to provide universal access to health care to all migrants was Thailand, which has also managed to keep its COVID-19 infection rate to a little over three thousand and the number of deaths to under sixty.[103]

The coronavirus has disproportionately affected migrant

workers—in the agricultural sector in Florida, in German slaughterhouses, in the construction industry in Singapore.[104] Many migrant workers have simply been pushed out: in the United Arab Emirates alone, more than fifty thousand Pakistani workers were repatriated while five hundred thousand Nepalese workers returned home from India.[105] These expulsions have helped spread the virus, leading for instance to a spike in infections in India's Kerala province, which hitherto had successfully flattened the curve.[106] The United States expelled twenty thousand people from the end of March to mid-May 2020.[107] "If you look at some of the data coming out of Guatemala, many people deported there from the United States arrived COVID-19 positive," reports journalist Todd Miller.

The economic consequences of expulsion have also been severe. "As people are being repatriated, sometimes involuntarily to their countries of origin, we're seeing wage theft in the form of unpaid wages or reduced wages for workers still required to work," notes Shikha Silliman Bhattacharjee of Global Labor Justice. "We may be seeing the biggest single historical moment of wage theft that we've ever seen globally."

The coronavirus crisis represents a moment of acute peril for everyone and thus an opportunity for solidarity, a sense that we're all in this together, citizens and non-citizens alike. "When the virus struck, we thought that this will be a moment for Western society to understand what we've gone through," points out Abdul Aziz Muhamat, an advocate for refugee rights originally from Darfur in northwestern Sudan. "We've seen the opposite: clashes between left and right, between 'us' and 'them,' the ones who are on the move with no place to stay."

Immigrants and refugees are leading efforts to change the system. In the wake of the Black Lives Matter (BLM) protests after the death of George Floyd—and calls to defund the police—some immigration advocates are amplifying more radical demands. "At the most fundamental level, the current capitalist system is a driver of a lot of the violence and inequality playing out at borders and in the way people on the move are treated," argues Reece Jones of the University of Hawai'i. "So, we can use these moments of disruption to talk about the larger structural issues, to question the state as this fundamental institution, and question the legitimacy of borders as normal."

Border Controls

More than 135 countries imposed some kind of border controls once the pandemic began to spread. Europe reestablished its internal Schengen Area borders for the first time in twenty-five years and closed its external borders to boot. Some countries—Japan, New Zealand—practically walled themselves off.

"Restrictions on cross-border movements are obviously going up, including bans on people coming in by airplane where they need visas for access," reports Jacinta González of Mijente on the situation in the United States. "But also people trying to cross at the southern border are not being able to get into the country to ask for asylum. The Trump administration already established those limitations, but it has used COVID-19 as an opportunity to apply them full stop."

The whole point of US policy over the last twenty-five years has been "to make people as vulnerable as possible, to put them in dangerous situations," Todd Miller says. "With COVID, it's an exacerbation of that: further fortifying a border that has been fortified in unprecedented fashion, putting billions and billions of dollars into fortification to prevent people crossing through safe places and forcing them into areas that are intentionally dangerous."

With the pandemic comes the additional danger of exposure to infection. According to the Remain in Mexico policy, implemented by the Trump administration at the beginning of 2019, asylum seekers who attempt to cross the border are returned to Mexico, where they must stay for the duration of their legal proceedings. In Mexico, Miller adds, the returnees "essentially live in refugee camps where they are crowded together and are unable to physically distance." The first cases of infection appeared in these camps at the end of June.[108]

Epidemics have frequently fueled anti-immigrant narratives. In 1916, a typhus outbreak prompted the creation of disinfection facilities at the US border that required incoming Mexicans to take baths in a mixture of kerosene and vinegar. Later use of Zyklon-B in fumigation chambers at the border eventually inspired the Nazis to adopt the same chemical for use in concentration camps. During the *bracero* program that brought Mexican workers to the United States in the 1940s and 1950s, border officials sprayed arrivals with DDT and other insecticides.[109]

"We're seeing something similar with Immigration and Customs Enforcement (ICE) disinfecting people in detention and processing centers and a lot of immigrants showing the side effects of the chemicals that they've been exposed to," notes Josue De Luna Navarro of the Institute for Policy Studies. Meanwhile, he adds, immigrants have to pass a medical exam to get to the next stage in the process. "During those exams, if you test positive for a certain disease or are unable to show that you have all the vaccinations, it could jeopardize the process. It's unclear how the United States will put COVID-19 into play in these exams to keep people out."

As the pandemic gathered force in Europe, Turkey announced at the end of February that it could not handle a fresh influx of refugees from Syria and was therefore opening its borders to Greece. "Three major European figures flew to the area to reinforce that this was an external security border of Europe," reports Brid Brennan, "and everything was going to be thrown at it to make sure that no refugees would pass that border. A free hand was given to Greece to use live ammunition on people who were still trying to approach by sea in small dinghies." Two people were killed at the Turkish border.[110] Because of these incidents, she adds, "the European population could get a graphic view of what the externalization of borders for Europe means."

Borders became more militarized during the pandemic. The United States, Peru, Colombia, Poland, and many other countries sent additional troops to their borders to prevent the undocumented from entering. Portugal deployed drones.[111]

Similarly, just before the pandemic hit, Italy extended its cooperation agreement with Libya to police the Mediterranean and send back all unauthorized vessels, with migrants and refugees ending up in Libyan detention centers that Pope Francis has compared to concentration camps.[112] This

European policy on migration whereby "safe pathways across the desert or by sea are blocked" amounts to a "necropolitics" that combines with "an intensification of Islamophobia and anti-Chinese racism," Brennan concludes.

"If you are European, you are part of this continent, your country will provide you with medical service," observes Abdul Aziz Muhamat. "But if you're a refugee, you are on your own: no shelter, no place to stay, no health services. If you die, you die. If you're still alive, you can stay alive until they come and pick you up."

For right-wing parties long advocating tough border restrictions, the pandemic has been a political opportunity. "People on the right tend to use crises to their advantage, to reimpose a new order," argues Reece Jones. "You see that with corporations profiting off new weapons to police and patrol the border. You see that with Trump adviser Stephen Miller, who has used the pandemic to put into place strict rules even for legal immigration that the Far Right wanted for decades but never had an opportunity to do."

The more aggressive anti-immigrant politicians have worked not only to prevent people from entering but also to detain and expel the undocumented. In the United States, Jacinta González reports, "there was a hope at the beginning that COVID-19 could be used to explain why detention is not needed, that it's detrimental to people's health and facilitates the spread of the virus. But throughout the entirety of the pandemic, ICE activity has continued. The use of mandatory detention expanded. The system continued to defend the need for brick-and-mortar buildings to hold people."

Surveillance

The United States has been central to creating a border-industrial complex, "which is at the intersection of border policing, militarization, and profit," says Brami Jegan. This system relies on very lucrative public-private partnerships. Between 2006 and 2018, for instance, ICE, Customs and Border Patrol (CBP), and the Coast Guard handed out more than 344,000 contracts for border and immigration control services totaling $80.5 billion.[113] The use of information technologies to track immigrants has long been an integral element of this system.

"Some of the same companies with contracts for data analytics from ICE, like Palantir, are now getting the same kind of contracts from the Department of Health and Human Services to monitor data for COVID," reports Jacinta González. "Palantir has contracts with health organizations but has also been doing global relief for a long time. They've been tracking changing patterns in mass movements of people. But it's also biometrics and facial recognition and mass data from data brokers like Thompson Reuters and RELX Group. The use of surveillance as a necessary tool at this moment normalizes it. It also normalizes the use of big data that fuels these analytic projects."

Market forecasters predict an uptick for companies developing new technologies at the border, like artificial intelligence, "to look at people's health information, to see where people have traveled, to break into their social media accounts," Todd Miller reports. "They're talking about 'lucrative opportunity' and 'astonishing growth.' We're looking at a worldwide recession, but this industry is led by big corporations forecasting this ability to make a lot of money. These companies also have a lot of say in many places around world, especially in Washington, DC, to influence congressmen and the committees that dole out money."

"Tech and data companies are often very good at marketing," reports Jacinta González. "Sometimes, they told police departments that they need military grade equipment. Now they're telling the public that an alternative to policing is this technology that is race-neutral and not as invasive and violent, which we know is a bald-faced lie. But there will be a lot of politicians—from far right, but also center and center left—that will want to see this technology presented as alternatives."

There's a lot of money to made in the world of detention as well. When he was detained in the Moria refugee camp in Greece, Abdul Aziz Muhamat remembers being shocked to see G4S, a private security firm headquartered in the UK: "I saw how they torture people, how they use their power to push refugees to the point where they have to use drugs to deal with all of the pressure from these private corporations."

Climate Change

In thirty years, according to the World Bank, climate change will push more than 140 million people to migrate within their countries.[114] By 2070, areas where one out of every three people are now living will become uninhabitably hot.[115] Climate change has been a push factor behind migration out of Central America, with droughts, hurricanes, and crop failures prompting people throughout the region to pull up stakes and move north.[116] Rising sea levels are forcing Bangladeshis off their land and into a precarious existence in the capital, Dhaka, or abroad.[117] Even in relatively temperate Europe, extreme weather events displaced nearly seven hundred thousand people between 2008 and 2019.[118]

"Many people have a climate-change dimension to their migration and mobility," explains Alex Randall of the Climate and Migration Coalition. "They experience climate change via the market and via the labor market. Prolonged drought will impact their livelihood, their ability to gain money from agriculture, so they'll seek non-farm work elsewhere, which usually involves a move from rural to urban."

Their movement will also affect the livelihood of their family. "In these situations," he adds, "most people are earning money in their non-farm job and sending back remittances to their family, which becomes an important part of the survival and resilience of the household they left."

The pandemic disrupted how people in rural areas have been coping with climate change. "It's a really difficult situation for the people who have moved and for those who have stayed behind," Randall continues. "Many people with jobs in cities can't work because of the lockdowns or because their jobs are just not possible during the pandemic. The flow of remittances has stopped. The families back home are without that income plus people are returning to areas that are potentially climate vulnerable, moving back into the most at-risk locations on the planet, areas that will be hit by drought, by flooding, which was part of their decision to move in the first place."

Like COVID-19, climate change is impervious to borders. "Border security is a misnomer," Todd Miller points out.

"It doesn't secure anyone. The border apparatus imprisons people as a solution to those problems. It's becoming evident that the border apparatus didn't stop COVID and won't stop climate change or a host of other issues."

Labor and Social Policy

More than half the world's immigrants are migrant workers: 164 million out of 258 million, according to a 2017 International Labor Organization estimate.[119]

These workers represent a little less than 5 percent of the global workforce, but they have suffered disproportionately because of the pandemic.[120] Tens of millions of migrant workers have lost their jobs, and those that have continued to work in fields and factories have been at heightened risk of infection. Bahrain, Oman, and Kuwait have surged to the top ranks of states with the highest per capita infection rates because of the spread of the virus in the communities of migrant workers that run the machinery of daily life in the Gulf states.[121]

The pandemic has had major implications for low-wage workers in export processing zones, many of them women with no employment security and little or no social safety net. "The widespread barriers to accessing basic resources, food, and housing arguably approaches a humanitarian crisis," Shikha Silliman Bhattacharjee explains. "This is what the deliberate cultivation of a disposable workforce looks like."[122]

COVID-19 has divided the migrant workforce into two categories: "locked in" and "locked out."

"On the one hand, we have migrant workers locked into employment, including essential workers, those who don't have the social safety net or the personal savings to opt out of risky work," explains Shikha Silliman Bhattacharjee. This category includes "supply chain workers, essential workers, construction workers, domestic workers. We see exposure to COVID without personal protective equipment. We are also seeing people literally locked into workplaces. Domestic and care workers are given the choice: either you stay within employer households or you can't work at all. Also, in countries that have government lockdowns such as India and Sri Lanka, factories have locked workers into compounds and, to maintain the health level of the workplace, prohibited movement in and out of the space."

"On the other hand, there are those locked out of employment because of lockdowns or a shift in supply chain demand," she continues. These workers have suffered from widespread hunger and malnutrition as well as the health consequences of not having access to work or being stranded between jurisdictions.

In the United States, undocumented workers don't have Social Security numbers, which means that they can't access medical insurance. When the pandemic hit, the undocumented were reluctant to go to hospitals. "Even though it was clear that the government wanted to provide COVID tests for free, we knew that any visit to a medical institution meant that there would be a lot of bills," Josue De Luna Navarro relates. "How can a big community be expected to be healthy and know who has COVID when we've never been able to go to a hospital or see a doctor? Those clinics where people can go to find help are understaffed and overflowing, so many people decided not to seek help. There's also a fear in our community of exposing immigration status to medical institutions."

Resource-stretched governments and hospitals have focused medical attention on COVID-19. "All the other health needs of refugees—tuberculosis, HIV, respiratory illnesses that are very severe and life-threatening—have been deprioritized," Brami Jegan reports. "Vulnerable communities are nervous about accessing COVID health care because they might be separated from families. Their families are a lifeline, so there's a fear in refugee and displaced populations of even putting up their hands to say that they might have COVID."

The situation inside refugee camps is particularly dire. "Refugees are forced to stay in small areas where staff are not allowed to come in and provide supplies for basic needs," reports Abdul Aziz Muhamat. "No health care system has been set up for refugees to access. In the Moria camp on the Greek island of Lesbos, the medical organization Médecins Sans Frontières is not allowed to go inside the center to check refugees. There are twenty-two thousand people stuck together in that small place. Imagine twenty-two thousand people in three lines to access their meals. There's no social distance. They're stuck in there like sardines. If one person gets the virus, it will just spread from person to person."[123]

Nor have governments addressed the additional economic challenges faced by migrants and refugees during the pandemic. In the United States, government stimulus checks didn't go to the undocumented. "The government's decision to rely on Social Security numbers and not Individual Taxpayer Identification numbers, which all undocumented have in order to pay taxes, primed our community for failure," Josue De Luna Navarro explains. The pandemic has served as a "reminder that this is what the system was meant to do. It's based on racism, on using immigrant bodies as dispensable labor. The government doesn't care if I'm infected and I infect my whole family and community and they all die. The people in power make a choice to leave us out."

Governments in general have been indifferent to the plight of migrants. "We're not seeing strong lenses on gender, labor, migration, and business accountability coming through in the state policies that we do see," points out Shikha Silliman Bhattacharjee. "Governments are not providing safety nets for the most vulnerable, which actually creates conditions that drive them further into forced labor, whether at construction sites in the Gulf, garment supply chains in Asia, or the type of domestic situations in the United States where people are not in any position to bargain over working conditions or state that they want to exit because they have no other options."

Movement Responses

The pandemic has further marginalized the already marginalized. "We've gone from safe haven to safe haven, and in between we've suffered a lot of abuse, unspeakable things that we try to explain, but it's so hard for people to comprehend," laments Abdul Aziz Muhamat. "We've been excluded from platforms where we could share some of our knowledge and be part of the solution. Before, we were half-excluded. Now, with COVID, we are completely excluded."

Migrants and refugees are urging governments and advocacy groups to "look with us, not at us," Brami Jegan says. "This has to be a strong invitation by migrant and refugee communities to be consulted, to be protagonists central to the solutions." The lack of consultation has only exacerbated racism globally. "Instead of seeing this as a class and labor issue, it has been turned into 'migrants don't understand the language' or 'they have weird cultural practices that make us all sick,'" she continues. "In Australia, the Muslim population was targeted as the reason for an outbreak of a few cases in Victoria because of Eid rituals" that mark the end of Ramadan fasting.

Still, a number of migrant-led organizations, such as the Transnational Migrant Program–Europe, have worked to bring migrant and refugee voices into the policy debate. Refugees and migrants have been integral to a campaign to demilitarize the European Union border organized by the Stop the Wall movement, which has rallied against the wall separating the West Bank from Israel. "We got ten thousand signatures to block the EU from using drone technology from Elbit, an Israeli defense firm, on the Mediterranean," reports Brid Brennan, who also notes "the extraordinary creativity and mastery of technology of the WatchTheMed Alarm Phone hotline developed by activists to support crossings of the Mediterranean. They've turned technology against the makers of technology."[124]

Another example of solidarity is the organizing taking place across migration corridors. "In India and Sri Lanka, trade unionists are working to make sure that workers in Jordan and other countries in the Gulf get up-to-date information on what's happening in the lockdowns in their own countries," Shikha Silliman Bhattacharjee explains. "Workers who were able to contact their families then had their families contact unions in home areas to coordinate."

After several months of shutdown, the Black Lives Matter protests in summer 2020 re-energized movement organizing. Some protests focused on the loss of migrant lives, like the gatherings in Britain that mourned the death in 2019 of a twelve-year-old Somali girl.[125]

"If you had told us six months ago that something like that would happen, we would have said it would be hard to envision," observes Reece Jones, adding that the movement morphed from challenging police violence to a more thorough questioning of white supremacy. "I can see how that kind of questioning of the entire foundations of the United States as a country could extend to the question of how the country fits into a global system of states, which are all based on a similar foundation of exploitation, of restricting access to resources, of allowing the capital class to control wealth and power."

At the same time, the undocumented have faced additional risks at these protests.[126] "The police have brought in the Drug Enforcement Agency, FBI, and ICE agents to retaliate against protesters," Jacinta González says. "That has a tremendously chilling effect on the way people are organizing during this crisis." The Border Patrol also joined the federal crackdown on protests in Portland, Oregon, in July, not to mention being deployed overseas in Iraq, Afghanistan, and elsewhere as part of "counter-terrorism" missions.[127]

Efforts to address the plight of migrants and refugees largely take place at a national level where advocates lobby for changes in immigration laws or the management of border security. But migration is a transnational issue.

"It's hard to think outside the presentism of our era to see the state as just a blip on the radar of human history," Reece Jones points out. "But using borders to divide the world in bounded containers of power is a new idea. Using these bounded spaces to control resources and institute power over other groups of people: that's the history of early states. The pandemic again raises the problem of the scale of the issues we're facing. These issues, whether climate change, migration, or the pandemic, are global, but we continue to think about these problems through this lens of states. That will always produce inadequate solutions."

Another tension in the movement to rethink borders and migration is between reformist measures like reducing the militarization of borders and more radical efforts like abolishing border policing agencies and eliminating borders altogether.

"If we abolish ICE and CBP and use the money for public health, we could provide two COVID tests per person or 718,000 COVID-19 hospital stays," says Josue De Luna Navarro, citing figures from the National Priorities Project.[128] "Abolishing the border industrial complex is not just the moral thing to do but it's good for our public health. We must really dismantle physical and technological borders and those systems put into place to kill our people—not only in the United States but where the United States has increased border threats around the world."

"Big ideas are great and they keep us moving," Jacinta González agrees. "But I'm also hesitant about conversations around very abstract demands that don't talk about how communities are empowered to get to those places. We're in a crazy moment in the United States where people are saying 'abolish police,' but police budgets are still going up. If people are talking about big bold ideas from protected places and are not having conversations with groups confronting xenophobia, police violence, and immigration enforcement on the ground, the possibility to push those ideas forward becomes distant. It has to be done with nuance and the relationship building that comes from walking the same path together."

Josue De Luna Navarro acknowledges the tension between the practical and the visionary. "Growing up undocumented, my sister was organizing to get a driver's license. So, she hears academics talking about no borders and she's thinking, 'I don't care, I just want my driver's license.'" At the same time, movements for abolition—of institutions like ICE, of borders more generally—understand "that the big goal of liberation is not about making immigration work for us," he continues. "This system is working how it was designed. It works only for those with privilege. There needs to be a balance like everything in life, a balance between being able to go to the hospital and have medical insurance and the big ideas like opening the borders."

That work is ongoing, Brid Brennan points out. "There's maybe a misreading of the mobilizations happening in the United States and in Europe as spontaneous. No, it's the fruit of years of work and strategizing and making roadmaps to where people want to go and the kind of transition they want."

Chapter 4: Rethinking Borders and Migration Discussion Participants

SHIKHA BHATTACHARJEE is a lawyer and the research director for Global Labor Justice (GLJ) in Washington, DC. She leads GLJ's work on labor migration in the Persian Gulf and Jordan.

BRID BRENNAN is the coordinator of the Corporate Power project at the Transnational Institute in Amsterdam. She is co-founder of the European Solidarity Centre for the Philippines and, most recently, RESPECT, a Europe-wide anti-racist network for migrant domestic workers.

JACINTA GONZÁLEZ is a senior campaign organizer at Mijente, based in Arizona, and an expert in organizing against immigration enforcement and the criminalization of Latinx and immigrant communities.

BRAMI JEGAN is a Tamil woman and activist in Australia. She works for the Global Strategic Communications Council, a network of climate communicators. She is working on a new project that aims to stigmatize corporate actors profiting from border policing.

REECE JONES teaches in the Department of Geography and Environment at the University of Hawai'i at Mānoa. His latest book is *Violent Borders: Refugees and the Right to Move.*

TODD MILLER is a journalist based in Tucson, Arizona, and the author, most recently, of *Empire of Borders: The Expansion of the U.S. Border Around the World* (Verso, 2019) as well as the TNI report, More than a Wall.

AZIZ MUHAMAT is a human rights advocate for migrants, refugees, and asylum seekers, based in Geneva. He is also the 2019 Martin Ennals Award Laureate for Human Rights Defenders and a UN fellow at the Office of the High Commissioner for Human Rights (OHCHR). He has worked as a social worker, journalist, advocate, and vlogger/podcaster, and an author in collaboration with other refugees offshore and inshore on Manus Island. Originally from Darfur in northwestern Sudan, he was held for six years in detention on Manus Island, Papua New Guinea.

JOSUE DE LUNA NAVARRO is the New Mexico Fellow at the Institute for Policy Studies. He is the founder of the national UndocuHealth program for United We Dream. In New Mexico, he is the co-founder of the New Mexico Dream Team (NMDT), the largest statewide undocumented-led organization in New Mexico. With the NMDT, he directed a research study in collaboration with the University of New Mexico's TREE Center for Advancing Behavioral Health regarding the health impact of anti-immigrant and racist policies on undocumented youth.

ALEX RANDALL is a leading specialist in the connections between climate change, migration, and conflict. He is program manager at the Climate and Migration Coalition, based in the UK. He has been working on issues around climate, migration, and human rights for fifteen years. He advises a number of key international agencies and governments on their responses to climate-linked migration and displacement. He has also served on the advisory group of the Nansen Initiative and Platform on Disaster Displacement. He has written extensively on climate change and migration for the *Guardian*, *Le Monde diplomatique*, *New Internationalist*, *Prospect*, and numerous other outlets. He is the author of a number of book chapters focusing on the connections between climate change and the rights of refugees and migrants.

BUDGET PRIORITIES

Military spending goes down when countries feel less of an overall security threat or more of an overall budget constraint. The novel coronavirus should exert a downward pressure on military budgets for both reasons. Abandoning current conflicts and squabbles, the world could be cooperating to fight a common enemy that can't be defeated with tanks or nuclear weapons. And the subsequent economic downturn has required bailout packages that have placed enormous debt burdens even on governments that entered the crisis with balanced budgets.

And yet, there's no indication of a substantial transfer of money out of the military. In 2019, global military spending rose 3.6 percent to more than $1.9 trillion, the largest spike in a decade.[129] Despite COVID-19, the major powers seem determined to set a new record in 2020.

The United States was leading the world in COVID-19 infections and deaths in summer 2020. Yet, at the same time, the Trump administration pushed for more money for the military with a $740 billion budget for the Pentagon's 2021 base budget, nuclear weapons, and overseas military campaigns.[130]

Goaded by the Trump administration to spend 2 percent of their GDP on their militaries, European members of NATO increased their spending by 10 percent in 2019. With the goal of reaching that 2 percent goal by 2025, France announced significant budget increases prior to the outbreak of the pandemic.[131] Poland, too, announced in January that its military budget for 2020 would register an 11.3 percent increase over the previous year.[132] Long after the pandemic hit, Hungary announced in July an astonishing 26 percent increase in military spending for 2021.[133]

China, the world's second-largest military spender after the United States, announced in May 2020 a 6.6 percent increase in its military budget, which, although significant, is also the smallest increase in over a decade.[134] Other countries, too, announced boosts in military spending: India (6 percent for 2020–21), Pakistan (nearly 12 percent for 2020–21), and Brazil (an unbelievable 48 percent for 2020).[135]

After increasing its military spending by 10 percent in the first six months of 2020, Russia announced in July that it would consider cuts because of budget constraints.[136] South Korea, too, announced a reallocation of over $700 million from the military to its COVID response (though its military budget for 2020 will still post a significant increase).[137] Such second thoughts are more the exception than the rule, however, at least until the bill for COVID-19 comes due.

Meanwhile, despite a plea from the UN secretary general for a global ceasefire, conflicts continued: in Afghanistan, Yemen, Syria, Ukraine, Myanmar, and elsewhere. Global arms sales, which fuel these conflicts and have risen steadily since the early 2000s, don't appear to have been adversely affected by the pandemic as leading exporters, like the United States, have rushed to facilitate new deals.[138]

In some cases, the pandemic provided a rationale to bail out the military-industrial complex. "France and Germany are putting more money into their arms industry to keep them going after the coronavirus crisis hit them hard," reports Wendela de Vries of the European Network Against the Arms Trade, "especially industries that also produce civilian airplanes where the market has collapsed."

The military's involvement in the campaign against COVID-19 reinforced an ongoing global turn toward authoritarianism. Philippines president Rodrigo Duterte, for instance, relied on the military to plan and implement the country's lockdown and has promised to use soldiers to distribute an eventual vaccine.[139] On top of that, Duterte pushed through a new anti-terrorism law in July 2020. "The new anti-terror law in the Philippines is worse than what it was during the martial law years," reports Corazon Fabros of STOP the War Coalition (Philippines). "It is a classic example of a government that tries to muzzle not only the press but people who are critical of its governance."

Democratic countries, too, relied on the military, with the US Army Corps of Engineers building emergency facilities to help overwhelmed hospitals and the UK's Defence Science and Technology providing the use of laboratories for public health research.[140] In Spain, the military touted its role in the COVID response, though its actual participation was relatively minor. "This was done as propaganda to legitimize the military, to say 'we are here to help the country and we need the military to help us in the future,'" notes Jordi Calvo of the Centre Delàs.

Although governments asked military industries, if only temporarily, to produce critical goods like ventilators, the track record has not been encouraging. But the pandemic has accelerated certain transformations within the military: from a reliance on personnel and fixed positions toward a greater focus on automation, the cyber realm, and outer space.

What the outbreak of the virus hasn't encouraged, however, is greater cooperation among international institutions, governments, or militaries. In fact, the world's two most powerful countries, China and the United States, have witnessed a sharp deterioration in relations. Yet, as William Hartung of the Center for International Policy points out, the two countries have "plenty of things to cooperate on: climate change, building up the World Health Organization, and dealing with the pandemic itself, be it developing a vaccine, producing a vaccine at scale, or distributing it fairly around the world."

In the end, the pandemic has suddenly and vividly demonstrated that all the money spent on the military has not protected the homeland. "We are in a revolutionary moment," suggests David Vine of American University. "We need to use President Eisenhower's language of theft to help others see that every dollar spent on the military is a dollar not spent on people lined up outside my door waiting for free food. We need to have a greater sense of urgency, a greater sense of transforming the world."[141]

Retooling the Military

The military devotes a lot of money to protecting its soldiers. Yet the pandemic made a mockery of these efforts when it infected more than 1,100 sailors on the aircraft carrier USS *Theodore Roosevelt* in March and April, killing one and sidelining the vessel.[142] There have also been COVID-19 outbreaks at US military bases at home and abroad, notably on Okinawa.[143]

Even before the pandemic hit, Pentagon planners were addressing the chronic vulnerability of personnel by expanding the role of automation and the use of robots. All branches of the military are investing in remote-controlled craft: not just drones, but also ships operated from shore, "large unmanned surface vehicles," and self-driving tanks.[144] Because of COVID-19, "there likely will be less desire to put US forces on the ground and more reliance on speed, whether through computers, killer robots, or fast weapons," notes Jeff Abramson of the Arms Control Association. "There will be an increased reliance in the military on things that happen quickly, whether in cyberspace or with quicker weapons like hypersonics. Much of that will rely on commercial research and development."

This greater reliance on artificial intelligence (AI), robotics, and drones "is a danger not fully addressed by the peace movement," William Hartung warns. "We talk about reducing the size of the forces, but with new technology the Pentagon could be just as interventionist only in a different form. It may even claim that this will save money, which I think is dubious."

The pandemic has also exposed the vulnerability of military bases and what the United States calls "forward defense."[145] The Pentagon increasingly worries about its "targetable footprint," which can now equally refer to exposure to an adversary's missiles or to an unforeseen virus. Concern about the former prompted the United States in spring 2020 to transfer strategic bombers from Guam back to the mainland.[146] Anxiety over the latter might lead to a drawdown of overseas personnel, inspired by the reduction of twelve thousand US soldiers from Germany in July 2020, half of them slated to relocate to the United States.[147]

In Europe, the pandemic has encouraged a trend toward greater military cooperation outside NATO. "European countries are drifting further from NATO," reports Wendela de Vries. "This is strengthened by the French-German initiative to have more European defense." Both countries have supported EU military cooperation—which, in July, was included for the first time in the EU's long-range budget—in part as a hedge against a wavering US commitment to transatlantic relations.[148]

On the whole, De Vries continues, "I have a feeling that it's very hard to influence what the military is doing. This feeling might be quite common in the general public. Maybe we should bring back the feeling that we have influence. In the 1980s, we forced them to have disarmament treaties, which are now breaking down. But those happened because of a strong public movement demanding another kind of policy."

Military-Industrial Base

Every major power maintains an industrial infrastructure to support the military. Those firms also manufacture for export, which not only brings in hard currency but also, because of economies of scale, reduces the per-unit production costs for domestic use. As Jordi Calvo notes, increased military spending correlates with increased arms exports as well as increased armed conflict. An increase in armed conflict in turn generates more military spending by the participating countries and an uptick in the arms trade. The global military-industrial complex continuously benefits from this feedback loop.

The pandemic has threatened the workforce that keeps this complex humming, and the subsequent lockdowns have also jeopardized some of this industrial base. "There's been an increased effort to sell weapons to keep the industrial base going," Jeff Abramson reports. "Trump in his rhetoric has done this more than anybody else. Obama did this too. Who knows if a Biden administration would really curtail this."

In the United States, the production of any given weapon is spread out across many districts to ensure congressional support. To maintain and expand this industrial base, defense contractors pitch the manufacture of missiles and jet fighters as jobs programs, which many politicians find persuasive, particularly at a time of high unemployment. Any challenge to the economic underpinnings of the military, then, will encounter "a lot of resistance from communities and congressional members whose district rely on these contracts for jobs," points out Lindsay Koshgarian of the National Priorities Project.

In Spain, even with a leftist government, "defense is untouchable," Jordi Calvo reports. "The proposals from the conservative parties in terms of military and defense are the same as those of the left parties. And there's an agreement between Podemos and the Socialist Party not to talk about defense." Spain's leftist government has portrayed military outlays as "social spending" that creates thousands of jobs.[149]

"The military industry is using employment as the main

argument, trying to convince us that it is important and needs public help," Calvo continues. Yet, many studies have demonstrated that military spending is relatively ineffective at job creation. In a 2011 report, the Political Economy Research Institute showed that a billion dollars invested in military spending produced far fewer jobs (11,200) than a comparable amount devoted to education (26,700), while a 2019 Watson Institute study projected an additional 2,000 jobs for every billion dollars shifted from military spending to Green manufacturing.[150]

Skewed budget priorities aren't just a problem for wealthy countries. In 2019, military spending in the Philippines increased by 22 percent, with an additional 9 percent increase projected through 2024.[151] Meanwhile, as Corazon Fabros points out, the Duterte government has dramatically increased the foreign debt, made the country even more dependent on food imports, and failed to create job opportunities for 2.2 million overseas workers. "These people are being dismissed because of the pandemic," she reports. "It's a big problem: there are no jobs waiting for them."

The failure of so many countries, the United States in particular, to contain the pandemic starkly exposes the magnitude of the funds wasted on the military sector. "This is a world-historic moment for profound structural change unlike any in our lifetimes, rivaled perhaps only by the end of the Cold War," notes David Vine. "We have to show how disastrous US industrial policy has been because it has been so dominated by government investments in arms and other military production. We need to make that argument to the corporations and capitalists that have not benefited from decades of massive investment in military industries and the transfer of wealth that this investment represents. We have to show them that to make the United States economically competitive in the twenty-first century, we have to shift money away from this disastrous military-focused industrial policy."

Guns to Butter

A little over a decade ago, the United States entered a recession after the global financial crisis, and the economy shrank by 2.5 percent in 2009.[152] The national debt increased as a result of deficit spending to bail out the economy. In 2010, US military spending peaked at $849 billion and began to drop—even though the recession, by that time, was over.[153] The military budget would fall to $662 billion in 2017, largely as a result of deficit reduction efforts, before beginning to rise again under Trump.

In 2020, the US economy is expected to contract by as much as 7 percent.[154] The bailouts this time have been larger, and government debt has risen higher as well. The guns-versus-butter debate will likely be much sharper than it was in the early 2010s, particularly since the pandemic has revealed important vulnerabilities in the social safety net.

"The public health system is underfunded, dispersed, and dysfunctional," William Hartung points out. "It has not been invested in to the degree that the military has. The Centers for Disease Control (CDC) gets one percent of what the Pentagon gets. State and local public health entities have gotten less and less support from the federal government." Indeed, the budgets of states and cities have plummeted as a result of the pandemic. "There will be huge cuts necessary because the vast majority of states don't have the option to borrow money," notes Lindsay Koshgarian. "Schools can't figure out how to reopen without help from the federal government. We can't put in the health interventions we need without the federal government. The anti–federal government view that we don't need the government except for the military is going to be really challenged."

In Europe, Jordi Calvo reports, "for the first time, many people are talking about threats to our security that are not just military. The pandemic appears in the national security strategy here in Spain, but it was last on the list. Now it is going up." In another positive sign, Spain closed its immigration detention centers because of COVID.[155] "Also, there's a big campaign to make regular the situation of the roughly five hundred thousand migrants, which was forbidden for a long time," he adds. "It's an indication that the conversation around budget priorities can make a change."

Given the challenges of cutting defense spending, notes Miriam Pemberton of the Institute for Policy Studies, "the temptation is to figure out how to get money for priorities such as climate change or breast cancer research *within* the military budget." In terms of beneficial civilian projects funded by the military, she points to the repurposing of the Los Alamos nuclear weapons lab, which initiated the mapping of the human genome and is now working on a COVID-19 vaccine. But, she concludes, "the temptation should be resisted in many cases because it becomes just another argument for a bigger overall military budget."

In the United States, military production is largely in the hands of private companies like Lockheed Martin and

Boeing, which dominate weapons contracting, and it's not easy to enlist their help in the fight against the coronavirus. "The companies that the US government used its authority to fund to produce ventilators or masks were not in the defense industry, compared to countries around the world where the defense industry is government owned and where they were better able to direct their defense industry to change," Jeff Abramson points out. "The Lockheeds of the world were not nimble enough to repurpose."

"Some of these big companies are dysfunctional," William Hartung agrees. "I don't know how much money we want to entrust to them for things that we need."

There are a few examples of conversion from military to civilian production, such as the Philadelphia Navy Yard, which now produces commercial tankers along with Green energy technologies and also hosts a gourmet restaurant and the Tastycake bakery.[156] "But there are not nearly as many examples of military contractors shifting over to civilian production as there should be," Miriam Pemberton laments. "What's required is a significant shift in federal budget priorities. This happened to a degree after the Cold War, and some contractors did successfully repurpose their military technologies. The hydraulic system of a fighter jet, for example, is now powering hybrid electric buses in several cities. A real pandemic pivot in the budget would push other contractors in similar directions."

Then there's the question of military personnel and outside contractors. On the active duty side, "converting members of military into an unarmed public health force would be a useful policy proposal," David Vine suggests. On the manufacturing side, William Hartung sees potential in persuading workers to support conversion. "There was some resistance in Silicon Valley to getting involved in military projects," he notes, referring to Google employees who successfully protested a Pentagon AI contract.[157] "If workers had options to do work that is well compensated, if not within the same company then in the same region, they wouldn't be tied to the military corporate system."

When workers at Lucas Aerospace in the United Kingdom faced possible layoffs during the recession of the 1970s, they came up with more than a hundred different socially useful products they could build instead of jet fighters.[158] Similarly, the UK's Coalition Against the Arms Trade (CAAT) is applying the Lucas model to the field of renewable energy. "A move towards offshore wind and marine energy could produce more jobs than the entire arms industry employs," CAAT concludes.[159]

"The climate movement here in Europe is saying: retrain workers in the fossil fuel industry," Wendela de Vries observes. "The same must be said for the military industry."

Multilateralism

The military budget not only has drawn away critical resources for human needs. It has also ensured that fewer funds are available for diplomacy.

In the United States, the annual budget of the State Department is a little over $50 billion. That is less than one-tenth of the Pentagon budget. In Europe, the gap is proportionately smaller but still wide (Germany, for instance, spends $50 billion on the military and $7 billion on the Foreign Ministry). Elsewhere, the gap can be even larger. India devotes about $2 billion to its Foreign Ministry but more than thirty times that to its military ($65 billion).

The diplomacy gap in the United States only reinforces the unilateral thrust of US foreign policy, which the Trump administration has amplified. As a result of its failures in addressing the pandemic at home and abroad, "the United States will be increasingly less relevant in solving problems internationally and in its own international security moving forward," predicts Jeff Abramson. "The Trump administration's response globally has been: you take care of yourselves and we'll take care of ourselves. The United States is increasingly perceived internationally as inept, and other countries are proving to be more reliable players in the international order."

The decreased relevance of the United States, Miriam Pemberton notes, "would be a good thing if it means a more multilateral, more internationalist foreign policy. I'm hopeful that Joe Biden will try to undo everything his predecessor did, particularly in this realm. It will be our job to push him toward more multilateralism and more internationalism."

The question is "will the United States age gracefully or try to bring the rest of the world down with it?" William Hartung says. "There's still a strong current here that the United States is and should be number one, which flies in the face of the bungling of the coronavirus. That will be a point of resistance to the better outcome, namely the United States as a team player in developing international cooperation without assuming that it will run the show."

When it comes to climate change or staying a member of the World Health Organization, a plurality of Americans favor a more globally engaged government.[160] But Trump's "America First" messaging has defined US trade and immigration policy, not to mention a more isolationist US foreign policy. Jeff Abramson worries about such messaging, like "America going it alone, America has to be self-sufficient, America shouldn't buy from China because they might spy on us. How do we counter these nationalist tendencies in both the domestic and international arena?"

In the COVID era, those nationalist tendencies have been felt with particular force in US-China relations. Trump's blaming China for the pandemic not only serves to deflect attention from his own failings but also feeds into the Pentagon's narrative of China as the most important military threat to US power. "The Pentagon was already pinning hopes on future funding on great-power competition," observes Lindsay Koshgarian. "The racist fear-mongering over the source of the pandemic and rivalry over vaccines and personal protective equipment have given that idea even more credence among Washington decision makers."

Human Security

Campaigns to "move the money" away from the military and toward human needs have been going on for several decades. The upward trajectory of global military spending, the steady increase of global arms exports since 2000, and the relatively few examples of actual conversion of arms manufacturing to civilian production all suggest that the campaigns have had limited success.

"Now we have the pandemic threat," Wendela de Vries

points out. "Also, climate change is much bigger than any military threat. But still money is invested in military research and fancier, high-tech military capabilities. Somehow, we are not able to get into this discussion about budget priorities. Is it useful to continue to have this discussion, or should we change the angle of discussion?"

The pandemic offers an opportunity to shift the discussion. "It is an opportunity to unite globally and transnationally given that people around the world are having a common experience," David Vine argues. "This is an opportunity to link movements across issues. Defunding the war on terrorism might be an easier ask because it's been such a clear disaster that very few people defend it these days. Defunding the Africa Command is also a great way to involve people interested in defunding the police and the military budget."

William Hartung agrees: "One challenge is to convince people that they can make a difference in addressing the power of the military-industrial complex. Some of the modest but real shifts the Black Lives Matter movement has made with respect to reforming/defunding/dismantling the police may be inspiring, at least to progressives."[161]

"The Movement for Black Lives has already called for defunding the military, has already made explicit connections between racism and the US military budget and militarism more broadly," Lindsay Koshgarian says, pointing to growing opposition to the Pentagon's 1033 program, which has supplied more than eight thousand law enforcement agencies around the United States with over $7.4 billion in decommissioned military equipment like rifles and armored vehicles.[162] But, she cautions, peace activists need to address their "lack of fluency in talking about race because it could very easily devolve into folks coopting the Black Lives Matter movement."

"The Black Lives Matter movement has been trying for years to make the abolition of police departments and the entire criminal justice system part of the debate," David Vine adds. "Now it's part of mainstream conversation. The same can be true for the military-industrial complex. We have to learn from BLM to ask for everything." In that light, he says, a bill introduced by Bernie Sanders (I-VT) in the Senate in July 2020 to cut Pentagon spending by only 10 percent "just seems bizarre and pathetic."[163]

"Originally I thought, 'Why aren't we asking for much more?'" Lindsay Koshgarian recalls. "From my point of view, a $350 billion cut is a starting point. The answer is: we need both. We need people saying $350 billion because if no one is saying it, it won't happen. But the ten percent call is smart: anyone who says no to it really is an extremist."

The Sanders bill lost 77–23.[164] "This is an extremely modest first step," William Hartung notes. "But the amazing thing is that there hasn't been a proposal like that in Congress that I can remember. We can't look to Congress to take the lead except for the most progressive members like Congresswoman Barbara Lee (D-CA). There's probably going to continue to be a gap between what the peace movement and Congress put forward until we have such a large movement that they'll lose their jobs if they don't take bolder actions."

The economic crisis, meanwhile, can cut both ways. Austerity politics can impose limits on military spending. "The last time deficit concerns came out on top, the Budget Control Act locked in the guns versus butter equation for ten years," remembers Lindsay Koshgarian. "We have to make sure things don't go in that direction again. On the other hand, depending on how the US presidential election shakes out, there could be another major stimulus bill, which could easily become a vehicle for a few tens of billions more in military spending if the contractors don't have enough opposition and before austerity kicks in."

Just as the Black Lives Matter movement has pushed the needle on policing, the climate movement has been able to effect change in the energy sector. The decision by BP in August 2020 to cut oil production by 40 percent and make a concerted effort to convert to clean energy might also inspire peace activists.[165] The international peace movement has indeed urged a shift from military spending to Green New Deals.[166] But, as Lindsay Koshgarian points out, the climate movement "is not as fluent as the racial justice movement in talking about the role of militarism. Climate activists have said, 'Why take on the Pentagon? We don't need another enemy.'

"The framework of just and equitable transition within the climate movement is too domestically focused," she continues. "It needs to be made more international. Once that happens, it would be much more natural for the climate movement to take positions on anti-militarism and the Pentagon budget."

In Europe, Wendela de Vries reports, "what we're trying to build up now with the climate movement is a focus on expeditionary forces—the big planes and ships that use a lot of fossil fuel and are used to control the world and protect the sea lanes to bring raw materials to the West for our consumption. It is one thing to have an army to defend your own country, it is something very different to have an army to defend your economic interests in someone else's country. We do not want fuel-consuming heavy armaments and transport capacity meant for dominating the world economy."

The pandemic has revealed the stark gap between military preparedness and medical preparedness. In spring 2020, the Global Campaign on Military Spending focused its annual actions on the spending disparities between health services and weapons, noting for instance that the budget for a single F-35 jet fighter could cover 3,244 intensive care unit beds while one battle tank translates into 440 ventilators.[167] "These actions were more successful than ever around the world," Jordi Calvo reports. "In Spain, there's also quite a big social movement that works only on health services and the budget. Health workers have long demonstrated in front of hospitals demanding more resources. They even inspired a political coalition during the past elections. Collaboration with such partners can help proposals to cut military spending."

Miriam Pemberton notes that, in the United States, "there's bipartisan enthusiasm for sixteen billion dollars for a national service corps for kids who are not able to go to college. What about proposing this as a public health force that's an alternative to military service?"

Budget priorities activists have other collaboration opportunities. "What is moving young people to go to demonstrations now is climate, refugees, and Black Lives Matter," Jordi Calvo notes. Also, peace activists have been "following boats where arms go to Yemen. When they stop in a Spanish harbor, activists demonstrate against the weapons. It's not a lot of people, but there's been coordination among Italy, Spain, and the Netherlands."

The challenge, Corazon Fabros explains, has been to

translate the information on military spending and budget priorities into materials "so that people really feel it, so that young people realize that their lives and futures are at stake."

The acute threats of the pandemic and climate change force a reevaluation of the very notion of security. Even if retooled on the margins to manufacture ventilators or run on clean energy, the military-industrial complex remains dedicated to building weapons, deterring military threats, and waging wars. In contrast, human security, which assesses all threats to well-being including risks to food, shelter, and health, provides a better framework for evaluating budget priorities. A recent statement by humanitarian disarmament organizations around the globe on the COVID crisis urges the world to "prioritize human security, reallocate military spending to humanitarian causes, work to eliminate inequalities, ensure multilateral fora incorporate diverse voices, and bring a cooperative mindset to problems of practice and policy."[168]

As William Hartung concludes, "The current system can't solve the problems we're facing. That's our opening to make the kind of constructive policy we want."

Chapter 5: Budget Priorities Discussion Participants

JEFF ABRAMSON is a senior fellow at the Arms Control Association in Washington, DC, and directs the Forum on the Arms Trade, an international network of more than eighty experts working to address the implications of the arms trade, security assistance, and weapons use.

JORDI CALVO is the vice president of the International Peace Bureau. He is an economist and peace culture, disarmament, and defense economy researcher. He is the coordinator of the Centre Delàs in Barcelona and is an armed conflicts, defense economy, and cooperation lecturer.

WENDELA DE VRIES is a longstanding researcher and campaigner on arms trade and the defense industry for Stop Wapenhandel in Amsterdam and the European Network Against Arms Trade, among others. She recently wrote *Hoe de wapenindustrie probeert te profiteren van de coronacrisis* (How the arms industry tries to profit from the corona crisis) and "Fossil Wars, Arms Trade, and Climate Justice," and is running the petition campaign Geen geld voor nieuwe wapens (No money for new weapons).

CORAZON VALDEZ FABROS is the vice president of the International Peace Bureau and a core member of the Peace and Security Thematic Circle both at the civil society process at the Asia Europe People's Forum and the ASEAN Civil Society Conference/ASEAN Peoples' Forum. She is lead convener of the STOP the War Coalition (Philippines) and Nuclear Free Pilipinas. She was the former chairperson of the Pacific Concerns Resource Centre (the secretariat of the Nuclear Free and Independent Pacific Movement) and the secretary general of the Nuclear Free Philippines Coalition (NFPC). She is a lawyer by profession, a founding member of the National Union of Peoples' Lawyers, and formerly a business administration professor at the Centro Escolar University in Manila.

WILLIAM HARTUNG is the director of the Arms and Security Program at the Center for International Policy in Washington, DC, and a senior adviser to the center's Security Assistance Monitor. He is the author of *Prophets of War: Lockheed Martin and the Making of the Military-Industrial Complex* (Nation Books, 2011) and the co-editor, with Miriam Pemberton, of *Lessons from Iraq: Avoiding the Next War* (Paradigm Press, 2008). His previous books include *And Weapons for All* (HarperCollins, 1995), a critique of US arms sales policies from the Nixon through the Clinton administrations. From July 2007 through March 2011, he was the director of the Arms and Security Initiative at the New America Foundation. Prior to that, he served as the director of the Arms Trade Resource Center at the World Policy Institute.

LINDSEY KOSHGARIAN is the program director of the National

Priorities Project (NPP), where she oversees NationalPriorities.org. Lindsay's work on the federal budget includes analysis of the federal budget process and politics, military spending, and specifically how federal budget choices for different spending priorities and taxation interact. Prior to joining NPP in 2014, Lindsay was a researcher at the University of Massachusetts Donahue Institute, where she conducted state and regional economic development studies.

MIRIAM PEMBERTON is an associate fellow at the Institute for Policy Studies in Washington, DC, and former director of the Peace Economy Transitions Project.

DAVID VINE is professor of anthropology at American University in Washington, DC, and a board member of the Costs of War Project. David is the author of several books about war and peace including a new book, *The United States of War: A Global History of America's Endless Conflicts, from Columbus to the Islamic State.*

THE GLOBAL CEASEFIRE

On March 23, 2020, UN secretary general António Guterres issued an appeal to the warring factions of the world to lay down their weapons and observe a global ceasefire. The coronavirus pandemic was gathering force in hotspots like China and Italy, yet wars in Yemen, Syria, and elsewhere showed no signs of abating. It was the first time in its seventy-five-year history that the United Nations had made such a plea.

"To warring parties, I say: Pull back from hostilities," Guterres said. "Put aside mistrust and animosity. Silence the guns; stop the artillery; end the airstrikes. This is crucial . . . To help create corridors for life-saving aid. To open precious windows for diplomacy. To bring hope to places among the most vulnerable to COVID-19."[169]

The appeal initially garnered support from seventy governments, two hundred organizations, and twelve parties to conflicts, including the Communist Party of the Philippines and the National Liberation Army in Colombia.[170] By the end of June, 171 member-states signed onto a General Assembly resolution drafted by Malaysia.[171] Despite early US opposition—over the inclusion of a reference to the World Health Organization—the Security Council unanimously passed a resolution on July 1 calling for a ninety-day "humanitarian pause" in hostilities.[172] It was an encouraging sign in a world overcome by disease and economic shock.

Some of the ceasefires inspired by the appeal have endured in fragile form, as in southern Thailand.[173] For the most part, however, declared ceasefires did not hold, and violence actually increased in some of the signatory countries. Fighting barely let up in Yemen, the government and separatists continued to trade fire in Cameroon, and the civil war in Libya escalated into a major regional conflict.[174] Violence increased as well in Iraq and Mozambique.[175] Oxfam called the world's response to the global ceasefire a "catastrophic failure."[176]

This failure of the global ceasefire to gain traction is only the latest sign that even a global pandemic can't stop the terrible cycle of violence within countries and between countries. Consider, also, that the effects of climate change are leading to greater conflict over land and resources rather than cooperation to address the underlying challenges to the environment.[177] Military force has failed to counter either climate change or COVID-19, and these threats in turn have failed to disarm military forces.

"The pandemic has shown the vulnerability of the earth very clearly," points out Lora Lumpe of the Quincy Institute. "There is a tremendous opportunity to make really clear the relationship between a stressed-out planet and the direct threat that has us all sheltering in place and the complete and utter failure of militarism not only to win the Global War on Terror but to advance our security."

The shift away from democratic to more authoritarian

governance in much of the world has contributed to undermining the chances for ceasefires to succeed. The more autocratic style of Ivan Duque, for instance, has made an enduring peace in Colombia more elusive, while the authoritarianism of the absolute monarchies in Saudi Arabia and the United Arab Emirates (UAE) has prevented any opposition groups or figures in those countries from mounting campaigns to stop the war in Yemen. "Increasing authoritarianism has been a global trend for many years," notes Bridget Moix of Peace Direct. "The response to the COVID-19 crisis by many governments has been an increasing crackdown and use of militarized government power to shut down the civil society space."

Another long-term trend has been the resurgence of ethno-nationalism, reflected at the state level (Make America/Brazil/China Great Again) as well as the sub-state level (in eastern Ukraine or parts of Myanmar). Such nationalism has militated against international cooperation (for instance, between the United States and China) if not encouraged actual conflict (for instance, within South Sudan). The pandemic has accelerated nationalist competition over scarce resources and to secure new arms export deals instead of encouraging internationalist cooperation for peace.

A critical issue in determining the success of a ceasefire is compliance. COVID-19 rather quickly divided the world into countries where citizens acted in the common good and those where cultures of selfish individualism or economic desperation undermined public health restrictions. In high compliance countries, "we learned that people tend to cooperate," reports Akira Kawasaki of Peace Boat. "Social distancing or accepting the lockdown of the economy is all about helping others. Of course, it's also about helping yourself, but in the context of understanding that you might harm others." Such a spirit of mutuality can help move a conflict toward resolution, but the populace in countries riven by conflict frequently experiences the kind of additional threats to livelihood that weaken appeals to the common good.

Even if it hasn't ushered in a new era of international cooperation beginning with a global ceasefire, the coronavirus is nevertheless altering geopolitics. "The world that we knew is gone forever," observes Michael Klare of the Arms Control Association. "Any of our strategies, thoughts, beliefs, and notions that might have once made sense are no longer valid because they applied to a world that is now gone. COVID-19 is reshaping the world or accelerating changes that were already underway: fundamentally and permanently."

Those changes can be glimpsed in larger geopolitical conflicts like the deepening cold war between the United States and China as well as in the changing public perceptions of internationalism and the utility of military force. Even as the global ceasefire fails to go into effect, it has reignited an important debate over guns versus butter as well as a conversation over the very process of peace making.

Ceasefires rarely succeed at first: only 20 percent manage to take hold.[178] But, according to peace researchers Jason Quinn and Madhav Joshi, a broken ceasefire can help lay the groundwork for eventual peace.[179] Women are a key part of that success.[180] "Of the ninety-eight peace agreements that were negotiated between 2000 and 2016, women's participation in civil society and in official peace processes ensured both that the peace agreement was signed but that it also included gender provisions," observes Christine Ahn of

Women Cross DMZ. "The key is the nexus between women official negotiators and women's peace movements."

The secretary general's appeal can be as effective in its failures as in its successes, particularly if the pandemic generates a new public understanding of global cooperation. "When an outbreak of the virus is bad in other countries, it threatens us just as badly as an outbreak here," notes Kate Kizer of Win Without War. "The virus will spread beyond borders. We live in an interconnected world. That creates an opportunity to build a case for international solidarity that did not exist before in the public psyche."

Geopolitical Push Factors

In an ideal world, the pandemic would not only have resulted in a global ceasefire. It would have led to an immediate transfer of funds from military budgets to the institutions fighting the virus. Active-duty soldiers would have put down their weapons and picked up masks and gowns to help out at hospitals and clinics. Military contractors would have shifted production from jet fighters to ventilators.

And, as the two most powerful countries in the world, the United States and China would have sat down to figure out how they could cooperate against this common threat.

Almost none of this happened. "There was an initial period in January and February when China, the United States, and other powers cut back on military operations to avoid exposing their forces to the virus," notes Michael Klare. "COVID also forced the United States to withdraw some of its ships from operational service, most notably the carrier

Theodore Roosevelt. But then, fearing that their adversaries would take advantage of the slowdown, the major actors (China included) seemed to ramp up their military activities to show that they wouldn't be hobbled by COVID. This was made explicit in the US case: demonstration flights of B-1s, B-2s, and B-52s over the western Pacific were said specifically to show that the United States was able to muster the full extent of its power despite COVID."

The United States under Donald Trump showed no special enthusiasm for the secretary general's proposal or for scaling back any of its military activities. "Even with Trump's belligerence toward the international community, it's very telling that other governments will use the fact that the United States is carrying out military operations as an excuse to continue doing what they are doing," notes Kate Kizer. "Other governments use the US selling weapons to human-rights-abusing governments as an excuse to sell weapons of their own."

"The US government is totally uninterested in doing anything about the global ceasefire," adds Medea Benjamin of CODEPINK. "And some countries that have signed the ceasefire are so hypocritical. Countries that are part of NATO and have troops overseas haven't said that they're going to pull out their troops."

The Trump administration has pushed for the withdrawal of US troops from the greater Middle East, which could play an important role in the success or failure of ceasefires in the region. But Trump has not followed through on his rhetoric. He hasn't done anything to stop the fighting in Syria or Libya, he has largely supported Turkey's military ventures in both countries, and he vetoed congressional legislation to end US logistical support for the Saudi-led war in Yemen.[181] Meanwhile, the administration's drone strikes in Afghanistan, Yemen, Pakistan, Syria, Iraq, and Somalia have continued under a greater veil of secrecy.[182]

In an equally aggressive way, the Trump administration has pursued a regime-change strategy toward Iran, withdrawing from the Iran nuclear deal and applying harsh sanctions to squeeze the Iranian economy. In 2018, Trump provided the CIA with new authority to intensify a cyberwar against the country.[183] To kick off 2020, he orchestrated the assassination of a top Iranian official, Qasem Soleimani, the head of the Quds Force in the Revolutionary Guard Corps, at the international airport in Iraq. During the COVID period, the administration brought in regime-change enthusiast Elliott Abrams as the new special envoy to the country. A number of mysterious "accidents" have taken place inside Iran, including an explosion at the Natanz uranium enrichment facility, which were likely the result of covert Israeli operations.[184] The United States and Israel have frequently teamed up to provoke and destabilize Iran, for instance creating a regional anti-Iran coalition anchored by Israel and Saudi Arabia.

An even more potentially destabilizing factor in geopolitics today is the deteriorating relationship between the United States and China. "The foreign policy establishment in Washington has reached a consensus that China must be prevented from ever reaching equality status with the United States," says Michael Klare. "To prevent that from happening, any means can and must be used, up to and including military force. They expect to prevail in warfare after the military buildup is completed with the use of conventional weapons, but they are prepared to use nuclear weapons, too. If it's necessary to wreck the global economy and global institutions in the process, that's also okay."

Klare sees this anti-Chinese agenda as a consensus position among Republicans, Democrats, and Independents, and so does Christine Ahn. "Not to say that the Biden foreign policy team will be a continuation of the Obama administration, but I see a lot of the same neoliberal hawkish centrist thinking from his campaign," she observes. "We know that the pivot to Asia was birthed during the Obama administration, which was all about containing China. What will it take to challenge that thinking?"

What had once been a spirited debate between those who favor engagement with China and those who support containment has largely disappeared.[185] "During the Obama years, some even believed in a G2 of the two great economies to solve the world's problems," Michael Klare continues. "That notion has been utterly crushed. The liberal elites have joined with Wall Street and everyone else in a drive to crush China at any cost."

Lora Lumpe disputes the notion of complete unanimity on the China issue. "I feel that we have many powerful allies who share a desire to prevent this slide to cold war—perhaps more powerful allies than on any other issue I've worked on," she says. "Silicon Valley is freaked out. They have business interests in China they want to pursue. Universities want to maintain the flow of full-fare-paying students. Scientists want to maintain research collaboration and contacts. Environmental organizations know that they need China's partnership. There is a large diaspora of influential Chinese Americans, including the Committee of 100. So, there is a divide in the elite."

For two decades, Washington had been absorbed in its "global war on terror," which has been eclipsed by the new focus on China. "But I don't think the global war on terror has completely wound down," argues Phyllis Bennis of the Institute for Policy Studies. "It has wound down enormously in terms of on-the-ground US troop involvement and certainly US casualties, which are down to near zero. That means that the wars are nearly invisible here. People have no idea that we are still fighting these wars."

"The global war on terror won't go away," responds Michael Klare, "but it doesn't really have impact on US society except in those communities where the Pentagon goes after young men and women to draft. The new cold war with China will affect American society in many ways, including conscription down the road because they don't have the manpower to fight China. And it will affect the pandemic response, because they will want to put money into fighting China, not rebuilding the United States."

The key geopolitical choice facing the United States and its allies thus boils down to whether to confront China or to cooperate, however selectively, on common threats like pandemics and climate change. And that choice will hinge on differing definitions of national security. "The notion that the biggest threat to the US people is not terrorism or China but climate change is a very popular notion these days," reports Phyllis Bennis. "But the only way we know how to describe climate change is as a national security threat, implying a military-style solution that fits the goals of the Pentagon. One of our challenges is how to broaden the widespread understanding of the primacy of climate in order to better respond to climate change."

Ending Conflicts

As the pandemic was gathering force at the end of February, the Trump administration announced a peace deal with the Taliban.[186] The United States pledged to withdraw troops in fourteen months as long as the Taliban held up their end of the deal by keeping groups like al-Qaeda out of Afghanistan and negotiating in good faith with the Afghan government. Ending the war in Afghanistan, which had dragged on for two decades, could have been a centerpiece of the global ceasefire, and the UN indeed supported the agreement.

But direct negotiations between the Taliban and the Afghan government didn't materialize. The Taliban doesn't consider the government in Kabul to be legitimate, and Kabul doesn't trust that the Taliban are interested in power sharing. In a series of reciprocal moves, the government released five thousand Taliban prisoners and the Taliban freed one thousand government forces.[187] But as ceasefires came and went, fighting resumed. By August, more than three thousand civilians had been killed or wounded since the signing of the February accord.[188]

"The Afghanistan example is where there seems to have been the most movement" in terms of the global ceasefire, notes Bridget Moix. "But the success of ceasefires always comes down to whether those who promise them can actually deliver at a local level and restrain fighting. In most conflicts today, control over armed groups is no longer centralized in formal armies and so the work of local peacebuilding continues to be the most critical element. But it doesn't receive enough attention or support." Local peacebuilding remains weak inside Afghanistan, and the pandemic has complicated matters by infecting as much as one-third of the population or ten million people.[189]

On the Korean peninsula, meanwhile, the conflict has been ongoing for even longer. The Korean War broke out in 1950, though inter-Korean hostilities actually began several years earlier. That war came to a formal pause in 1953 with an armistice. "The peninsula has been under a ceasefire for nearly seventy years, and it hasn't stopped the massive militarization of the peninsula and the Northeast Asian region," observes Christine Ahn.

Donald Trump and North Korean leader Kim Jong Un met three times in an attempt to break the deadlock over North Korea's nuclear weapons program and US economic sanctions against the country. Although Pyongyang declared a moratorium on the testing of nuclear weapons and long-range missiles and the United States canceled some military exercises in the region conducted jointly with South Korea, the talks didn't produce a lasting agreement.

The pandemic initially hit South Korea hard, but the government successfully contained the outbreak without a full shutdown of the economy. North Korea, meanwhile, announced its first case of the disease at the end of July, though COVID had likely entered the country well before.[190] Pyongyang is enforcing strict quarantine, travel, and border restrictions.

"Still, the pandemic is creating other opportunities, such as the urgency to advance humanitarian aid to North Korea," Christine Ahn continues. "South Korea, for example, announced in August that it will donate ten million dollars' worth of humanitarian aid to North Korea through the World Food Program. The UN Security Council approved the South Korean–based Inter-Korean Economic Cooperation Research Center request for sanctions exemption to send ten thousand virus test kits to Pyongyang."

In response to the pandemic, the Northeast Asian region engaged in some information sharing and early warning, reports Akira Kawasaki. "It is notable that the South Korean government took a significant step in April to reduce military spending to provide compensation for people in the pandemic," he notes. "Japan has not declared any such steps, although it is supportive of the secretary general's call for a global ceasefire. The prospect of future budgetary limitations formed the background of the Japanese defense minister's decision, in June, to cancel the deployment of the Aegis Ashore ballistic missile defense system."[191]

At the end of January, the Trump administration unveiled its "peace plan" to resolve the conflict between Israel and Palestine, but it was effectively dead on arrival because it authorized annexation of Palestinian land and recognition of illegal Israeli settlements, did not call for a just solution for Palestinian refugees, or provide actual sovereignty for any non-contiguous Palestinian entity that might emerge in the future.[192] As a result, the Palestinian Authority cut ties with both Israel and the United States. "The early months of the pandemic saw increased 'security' collaboration between the Israeli military and the Palestinian authority in the West Bank, including some minimal medical support," reports Phyllis Bennis. Meanwhile, "cooperation in COVID testing between the UAE and Israel gave political cover for public engagement just before the announcement in August of new diplomatic ties between the two countries."[193]

In the end, the Palestinians have been even more isolated

than before in the West Bank and Gaza but also in the diaspora. That includes the 475,000 refugees in Lebanon, which faces a rising number of COVID cases on top of political paralysis, economic freefall, and a horrific accidental explosion in Beirut in early August.

Yemen, in the midst of what the UN has called the world's worst humanitarian crisis, is the country that arguably needs a ceasefire most. The war between Saudi-led forces and Houthi rebels has left over one hundred thousand people dead.[194] Famine and cholera have killed tens of thousands more. More than three million people have been displaced by the fighting, with another hundred thousand displaced since the beginning of 2020.[195] The pandemic threatens to magnify the suffering to an unprecedented degree. Yemen has only seven hundred intensive care unit beds, and 20 percent of the country's districts have no doctors at all.[196] According to one UN official, "The worst-case scenario—which is the one we're facing now—means that the death toll from the virus could exceed the combined toll of war, disease and hunger over the last five years."[197]

"COVID-19 has made the world's worst humanitarian crisis even worse," reports Medea Benjamin of CODE-PINK. "UNICEF has reported that there are now 2.4 million children that could face malnutrition by the end of 2020 if conditions don't change. Adding to the crisis is the cutoff of US funds.[198] It is unconscionable for the United States to cut off humanitarian aid to Yemen in the middle of the COVID-19 pandemic—especially after supporting the bombing of Yemeni hospitals." The Saudi coalition has exacerbated the problem by maintaining an air, land, and sea blockade, which has cut off all commercial imports into the country and exports from the country.

When there has been pressure from the outside, particularly from the US Congress and grassroots activists, the warring parties have been motivated to negotiate. "The new Democratic Party platform and Democratic presidential nominee Joe Biden have pledged an end to US support for the Saudi-led war," Benjamin adds. "There is also a growing chorus of civil society groups and congressional members calling for a restoration of USAID funding to Yemen."

Sanctions, particularly on arms sales, are one tactic to smother the fires of conflict. But they are difficult to maintain, are undercut by illicit deals, and often have limited impact.[199] Frequently, a country like the United States will use economic sanctions to punish adversaries—hurting civilian populations, not governments—rather than use sanctions on arms sales to end conflicts, for instance, maintaining punitive economic measures against Iran while allowing an $8 billion weapons sale to go through to Saudi Arabia despite its abysmal human rights record and leading role in the war in Yemen.[200]

"The pandemic has provided something of an opening on the issue of sanctions because new people have come out and said that sanctions are cruel," notes Medea Benjamin. "But we don't have a Congress that cares about this. There's nowhere to take the empathy that people have and the anger at what the United States is doing with these economic sanctions and put it into something that could be effective policy-wise."

A New Internationalism

The United Nations once represented a new internationalism: a better version of the failed League of Nations, a welcome alternative to the violent nationalism of World War II, a forum for global cooperation even during the bipolar struggles of the Cold War. In addition to negotiating accords that restrain the production and proliferation of weapons, the UN has been instrumental in promoting, monitoring, and policing ceasefires. Today, the UN runs thirteen peacekeeping operations in such places as Kosovo, Cyprus, Congo, South Sudan, and between India and Pakistan.[201] But in the last decade, it has been occupied more with closing down operations (Haiti, Liberia, Timor-Leste) than in establishing new missions.[202]

The Trump administration's decision to stop paying for peacekeeping hasn't helped matters. The United States is over $750 million in arrears just to the UN peacekeeping budget.[203] Lack of financing is arguably less important, however, than lack of consensus. Geopolitical conflicts among the great powers, which contribute to paralysis in the Security Council, prevent the UN from acting with greater authority and efficacy in separating combatants. The "global ceasefire," for all the rhetorical support it garnered from UN member-states, has also fallen victim to these geopolitical disagreements and fiscal deficits.

"The global ceasefire effort held promise but may become just another statement by the UN secretary general without enough traction, teeth, or active organizing behind it," says Bridget Moix. "There was a moment when the pandemic was creating a 'great pause' in the world, where a call for ceasefires made sense to a lot of people, but I think that moment has largely passed and we are now in the living-with-the-disease phase trying to figure out how to control it. I don't know that communities currently caught up in most conflicts would say that the call for ceasefires has improved their lives yet. If there had been a major movement organized behind the ceasefire effort, it would have had more impact and potential."

Akira Kawasaki agrees: "Civil society needs to strengthen the pressure on the governments to take concrete action, including cutting military spending and addressing the needs of affected people in conflicts."

The United Nations has always served two different functions. The Security Council still represents the World War II victors and, more generally, the interests of the great powers, the United States chief among them. But in its declarations and many of its institutions, the UN also represents the popular sovereignty of democracy and human rights. In this way it can function either as the instrument of an internationalism of the powerful or an internationalism of the many.

The United States plays a key role in determining which internationalism the UN will embody. "Just because the United States is pulling out of the WHO and the Human Rights Council and doesn't pay dues to the General Assembly doesn't mean that it won't put all the pressure that it always has on countries for not toeing the US line," Phyllis Bennis points out. "Declarations are fine but they don't have the enforcement capacity, especially when the United States refuses to even sign them. The UN shouldn't be 'a tool of American foreign policy' as Madeleine Albright called it. It has the potential to be a tool of internationalism, but we have to fight every step of the way to make it that."

This fight requires a broadening of the usual understanding of foreign policy as the domain of Washington policymakers and opinion shapers. "Our foreign policy, like our domestic policy, has been rooted in the dehumanization of Black and Brown people," says Kate Kizer. "That's a key reason why the United States favors the use of violence to address security threats, which results in killing and not in security for any community. This dehumanization offers a powerful opportunity to break down barriers between foreign policy and domestic policy and bring other movements into this conversation. If we're going to have transformational change—to make our visions a reality, push back against the anti-China narrative, and prevent militarization to the east—we have to bring other people into this analysis, so they understand that their struggle for their domestic priorities and liberation is tied up with the liberation of others around the world."

The relative decline of US power may well open up other opportunities. "People all over the world are expressing pity toward the United States for all the coronavirus deaths, and they have been joining solidarity demonstrations after the death of George Floyd," notes Medea Benjamin. "They are recognizing how flawed the US system is and that they should not look to the United States for global leadership."

One indication of this altered perception of the United States is the way that humanitarian organizations are treating the country. As Phyllis Bennis points out, "For the first time Médecins Sans Frontières is working in the United States in the Navajo Nation, because people there are desperate and don't have any other access to medical services."[204]

Meanwhile, Medea Benjamin points to the example of Cuba, which "has shown what a small, poor, blockaded country can do to show solidarity with the world. It spends a twelfth per person what the United States spends on health care, and it has managed to keep people inside the country safer as well as send brigades of health workers to work in thirty countries."

As the challenges encountered by the global ceasefire have demonstrated, peace can't be declared or imposed from above. It requires the active participation of all the actors on the ground—and not just the leaders of the warring factions.

"Change has to be led by those most impacted," Bridget Moix concludes. "Whether that's local communities in east Congo affected by violence there, or people experiencing the sharp end of US weapons hitting their communities, or communities suffering here in the United States. How do we create the space and organizing that allows for that change to happen more often?"[205]

Chapter 6: The Global Ceasefire Discussion Participants

CHRISTINE AHN is the executive director of Women Cross DMZ, a global movement of women mobilizing for peace in Korea. Based in Hawaii, she's also the co-coordinator of the global feminist campaign Korea Peace Now! Women Mobilizing to End the War.

MEDEA BENJAMIN is the co-founder of the women-led peace group CODEPINK and the co-founder of the human rights group Global Exchange. She has been an advocate for social justice for more than forty years. Described as "one of America's most committed—and most effective—fighters for human rights" by *New York Newsday*, and "one of the high-profile leaders of the peace movement" by the *Los Angeles Times*, she was one of one thousand exemplary women from 140 countries nominated to receive the Nobel Peace Prize on behalf of the millions of women who do the essential work of peace worldwide. Her most recent book, *Inside Iran: The Real History and Politics of the Islamic Republic of Iran*, is part of a campaign to prevent a war with Iran and instead promote normal trade and diplomatic relations.

PHYLLIS BENNIS directs the New Internationalism Project at the Institute for Policy Studies in Washington, DC, focusing on the Middle East, US wars, and UN issues. In 2001, she helped found and remains active with the US Campaign for Palestinian Rights. She works with many anti-war organizations, writing and speaking widely across the United States and around the world as part of the global peace movement. She has served as an informal adviser to several top UN officials on Middle East issues and was twice short-listed to become the UN special rapporteur on human rights in the Occupied Palestinian Territory. She has written and edited eleven books. Among her latest is *Understanding ISIS and the New Global War on Terror: A Primer*, as well as the seventh updated edition of her popular *Understanding the Palestinian-Israeli Conflict*.

AKIRA KAWASAKI is an executive committee member of the Tokyo-based NGO Peace Boat and an international steering group member of the 2017 Nobel Peace Prize–winning International Campaign to Abolish Nuclear Weapons (ICAN). He also serves in the Northeast Asia regional secretariat of the Global Partnership for the Prevention of Armed Conflict (GPPAC).

KATE KIZER is the policy director at Win Without War in Washington, DC. She has nearly a decade of experience working on human rights, democratization, and US foreign policy in the Middle East. Kate previously served as the director of policy and advocacy at the Yemen Peace Project and as US advocacy officer for Americans for Democracy and Human Rights in Bahrain.

MICHAEL KLARE is the Five College professor emeritus of peace and world security studies, and director of the Five College Program in Peace and World Security Studies (PAWSS) in Massachusetts. His books include *Resource Wars* (2001), *Blood and Oil* (2004), and *The Race for What's Left* (2012). His articles have appeared in many journals, including *Arms Control Today, Bulletin of the Atomic Scientists, Current History,*

Foreign Affairs, Harper's, the *Nation, Scientific American,* and *Technology Review.* He serves on the board of the Arms Control Association and advises other organizations in the field.

LORA LUMPE is the CEO of the Quincy Institute for Responsible Statecraft (QI) in Washington, DC. Prior to joining QI, she was an advocacy director at the Open Society Foundations (OSF), combatting the corrosive effects of militarism on democracy in the United States and abroad. She is an expert on several aspects of US hyper-militarization, including military budget, arms industry, weapons sales, military aid and training, child soldiers, gun running, and munitions with disproportionate impact on non-combatants. Prior to OSF, Lora worked for several progressive research and lobby organizations, including the Federation of American Scientists, the Peace Research Institute of Oslo, and the Friends Committee on National Legislation. She has worked on or led a half dozen humanitarian disarmament campaigns—from chemical weapons to cluster munitions. Her books include *Running Guns: The Global Black Market in Small Arms* (2000), *Small Arms Control: Old Weapons, New Issues* (1999), and *The Arms Trade Revealed: A Guide for Investigators and Activists* (1998).

BRIDGET MOIX serves as Peace Direct's US executive director in Washington, DC. She has worked for twenty years on international peace and conflict issues, with a focus on US foreign policy. Prior to joining Peace Direct's staff, she was part of its founding US board for four years. From 2013 to 2015, Bridget served as atrocity prevention fellow with USAID's Office of Conflict Management and Mitigation. She spent nine years lobbying on US foreign policy and peace issues with the Friends Committee on National Legislation, where she developed and led the Peaceful Prevention of Deadly Conflict program. She has also worked with the Quaker United Nations Office, Oxfam America, American Friends Service Committee, and the World Policy Institute. Bridget directed the Casa de los Amigos in Mexico City, a Quaker center of hospitality and international understanding, from 2006 to 2008. She also worked in Cape Town, South Africa, with the Quaker Peace Centre during her graduate studies internship. Her book *Choosing Peace: Agency and Action in the Midst of War* describes how local and global peacebuilders can work together.

INTERNATIONAL CIVIL SOCIETY

The first response to the COVID-19 pandemic was to avoid physical contact with other people and maintain "social distance" to reduce the risk of infection. Then, as the disease spread, many governments issued shelter-in-place orders, even curfews. Gathering with others to protest in public spaces seemed like the last thing that anyone would do.

But protests happened anyway.

First came the protests against government measures to contain the pandemic. Anti-lockdown demonstrations took place in several US cities, often at state Houses and often presided over by members of armed militias. Similar protests—featuring anti-vaccine slogans and xenophobic conspiracy theories—took place in Europe, Russia, and Latin America as well.[206]

Anti-authoritarian protests also broke out—in Israel, Mali, the Philippines—aimed at leaders who'd taken advantage of the coronavirus to consolidate their power.[207] Other protests, particularly those in the Global South fueled by anger over economic inequality and corruption, seemed to be an extension of the wave of demonstrations that took place in 2019, a year of unprecedented mobilization against austerity and autocracy.[208]

Even with all of this public protest in the middle of a pandemic, the street actions that spread in the wake of the police killing of George Floyd in Minneapolis on May 25, 2020, stood out for the intensity of the activism, the rapid global spread, and the immediate impact on society. Statues associated with racism and colonialism were toppled. Certain names, traditions, and products—Aunt Jemima and the Washington Redskins in the United States, Zwarte Piet in Belgium and the Netherlands, skin-whitening creams in India—were ignominiously retired.[209] Defunding the police became a mainstream concern.

The Black Lives Matter (BLM) protests against police violence took place throughout the United States, even in relatively conservative areas.[210] They also inspired nearly twenty thousand people to demonstrate in Paris, ten thousand demonstrators in Amsterdam, tens of thousands in Auckland, thousands in London and Berlin and throughout Australia. Protesters in Kenya and South Africa hit the streets to criticize police violence in enforcing pandemic restrictions.[211] Demonstrations in Latin America targeted police impunity in incidents of racial violence against citizens of African descent.[212] In Southeast Asia, minority groups challenged majority privilege.[213]

"Despite some of the hardest moments that we're going through, all the crises we're experiencing, people understand the power of collective action," says Cathy Feingold of the AFL-CIO. "There's a real hunger out there for movement building right now, and we're seeing it all over the world."

The BLM protests in particular underscore a central fact about the new pandemic era: a return to the previous status quo is impossible. "There is no going back to normal, whatever normal is," observes Cindy Wiesner of Grassroots Global Justice. Before the pandemic hit, people were on the streets protesting insufficient health care, police brutality, authoritarian politics, and economic inequality. COVID-19 only made these social problems more visible and more infuriating to more people.

Whatever barriers the pandemic placed before activists mobilizing at a national level, the challenges to organizing internationally have been even greater. Travel restrictions meant that international meetings of activists ground to a halt. Strategizing moved online, but not everyone in the world has access to high-speed Internet, and organizing by Zoom poses its own difficulties. Many groups that had previously participated in global gatherings like the World Social Forum (WSF) have refocused on national and even local priorities.

"Now we can't get people together just like after 9/11," points out John Cavanagh of the Institute for Policy Studies. "The World Social Forum was wonderful in busting us out after 9/11, and we're going to miss that for a couple years."

In this new era, international civil society faces a number of questions. What form will international organizing take in a time of pandemic? What are the appropriate targets for collective action at the global level? Who will be the agents of change and who will be the leaders of the new movements?

In one respect, at least, the pandemic lays the groundwork for a new kind of internationalism. "Despite enormous differences in terms of class and inequality, and between north and south, there is a sense of a shared experience," observes Edgardo Lander of the Universidad Central de Venezuela. "This recognition that people in the United States are facing problems similar to those faced in China, Italy, Spain, India, and Brazil opens a shared possibility of working together and recognizing what our common problems are."

No Going Back

The pre-pandemic world, for some, was a paradise of regular paychecks, regular trips to sporting events and bars, and regular get-togethers with friends and family. Their fervent desire for COVID-19 to disappear and for life to return to "normal" is not surprising.

But the time before the novel coronavirus was not exactly a paradise for everyone.

"There is no normal to go back to because normal wasn't good for working people around the world," says Cathy Feingold. "The global economy is based on labor arbitrage and environmental degradation, not rights and protections. It's also been a model based on informality and exclusion. We need a whole different model."

The pandemic has functioned like an x-ray, Cindy Wiesner points out, that reveals underlying problems that will be difficult to unsee: "There are sectors of people, primarily working-class, Black, Brown, Indigenous women, that are considered basically disposable in the name of maintaining the system. The reformist, neoliberal frames for solving these problems are not going to work. No incremental changes, no sense of tinkering will resolve these crises."

The pre-pandemic world was abnormal because of the rapid global warming of climate change. It was full of war and wasteful military spending. Migrants and refugees were crowded into miserable internment camps or forced to attempt dangerous trips to safe havens. None of this has changed, or else it has changed for the worse.

Many government responses to the pandemic have only added to these problems. "Stay at home, wash your hands, maintain social distance—these are simply not viable for many people in the Global South," notes Edgardo Lander. "In South America, where sixty percent of the labor force works in the informal economy with no social security and no unemployment insurance, to stay home means not to have an income."

The failure of so many countries in the Global North to contain the pandemic has changed how some potential immigrants view what's "normal" in the world of the wealthy. "People from Senegal, they were ready to migrate or die," observes Coumba Touré of Africans Rising. "But now they see people in Italy struggling with COVID in a way they didn't know was possible. They see that something is broken in capitalism and whiteness and Europe. This is the moment when alternatives should be stronger. We should be able to say, 'There are other possibilities. Some of them are under your nose that you don't see or care about.'"

Prior to the pandemic, the Far Right provided an alternative to the liberal mainstream and its conception of normal. "There's been a dance between a liberal establishment, which continues to exert some real force in places such as Brussels, and the neo-fascist Right," explains David Adler of the Progressive International. "That dance requires the former to point to the latter as an existential threat, as a justification for their clearly failed policies of the past thirty years, and the latter to point to the former as a hapless establishment driving the Right's sense of legitimacy."

The pandemic has shaken up the dance floor. In countries like Brazil and the United States, this radical Right has demonstrably failed to manage COVID-19. "Both Trump and Bolsonaro are likely to be tossed out," notes John Cavanagh. "In the United States, Trump will be replaced by the discredited liberal establishment, which nobody is enthusiastic about. It might be a landslide, which shows how much people hate Trump. We need a complete rejection of Trump, not just because he was terrible on the pandemic but because he was terrible on economic and social issues."

The rejection of both the neoliberal status quo and the far-right challenge will require progressive alternatives not just nationally but globally as well. "We seem resigned to the notion of the international space as decayed and disordered," adds David Adler. "We need to reimagine the international. We need to revive the international as a space of creative policy and institutional thinking."

Protest

The pandemic has revealed many vulnerabilities: in the health sector, the social safety net, democratic governance. But COVID-19 also revealed "an added vulnerability of the powerful," points out Coumba Touré. "There used to be a category of people untouchable by almost any harm. Of course, disease and death comes for everyone, but they used to be so privileged and now they were exposed, with the same vulnerability to the pandemic as the rest of us." Both Bolsonaro and the UK's Boris Johnson contracted the disease. The president of Burundi likely died from COVID-19.[214]

The pandemic has also thrown the economically privileged into a panic. "It's the first time that you see business leaders actually scared," Cathy Feingold notes. "We've had more joint statements with the International Chamber of Commerce than I've seen in my lifetime. The next step is to see businesses working with labor to put commitments made in these statements into practice."

The combination of social vulnerabilities and the sudden vulnerability of the powerful contributed to an upsurge in protest. The mobilizations around Black Lives Matter inspired others around the world to challenge the most powerful representatives of the state: the police and the army. The residents of the Kibera district of Nairobi, for instance, have faced a spate of extrajudicial killings by the Kenyan police.[215] "People who worked on this issue would write down the names of the people killed and put the list in a desk in the hope that someday someone would listen," Coumba Touré reports. "Now, they feel strong enough to speak about it and have the Kenyan government hear them."

This same combination of outrage and opportunity brought thousands onto the streets of Bamako, the capital of Mali, to protest the corrupt, autocratic policies of Ibrahim Boubacar Keïta. The protesters, who have also been fed up with the deteriorating economic and social situation in the country, have faced not only the risk of infection but of being shot with live ammunition.

"Yet, they come out every Friday, massive numbers of people

that nobody can contain," Coumba Touré continues. "But then what, once this president steps down? Many protesters are saying that their president is just a puppet of France. And once the president is out, he'll be replaced with another person in the same system. That's where we're stuck. Even in Africans Rising, as we invite pan-African solidarity with the people of Mali, we wonder how we can support and make real change happen." When the military ousted Keïta in August, the coup leader was indeed someone from inside the system who'd worked closely with and received training from the US military.[216]

At all levels—local, national, regional, international— civil society organizations help to organize protest, shape the demands of protesters, and translate those demands into public policy and political change.

But not all protests come from the left, and civil society is not always progressive.

"There are sectors of international civil society that are fronts for governments and elites, or are not internally democratic," points out Leo Baunach of the International Trade Union Confederation and Global Unions Washington Office. "We need to refocus on a better world with a new social contract, and what it will take to get there. Right now, that means fighting for material wins that rebuild communities by saving and improving lives."

Organizing Strategies

The pandemic has challenged the capacity of organizations across the board, from social movements all the way up to international institutions like the World Health Organization.

"All of us in movements are in both sprints and a marathon, and we're struggling to do both in this time of crisis," observes Cathy Feingold. "I'm worried that our movements will be exhausted. We have pretty weak capacity right now. The labor movement is being pulled in all directions. We're trying to figure out food banks, how to get masks to people, how to organize in the meat and poultry sector, how to get occupational safety and health standards passed—everything at the same time. And we're also facing massive layoffs of our members!"

At the multilateral level, for instance, the international labor movement is lobbying for comprehensive debt relief for countries during the pandemic as well as to reform multilateralism.[217] "People around the world understand that a reason why they do not have access to health services, social protection, or safe jobs, is because of the failed policies promoted by the international financial institutions," explains Leo Baunach. "We have to build movements capable of changing and challenging the international economic and political architecture."[218]

Increasingly, the pandemic has pushed organizing into the digital sphere. "This will undoubtedly increase the political power of the main social media corporations like Facebook," points out Edgardo Lander, "which will decide on their own without any democratic control whatsoever which political discourses are legitimate and which are not, taking the privatization of the public sphere to new levels and severely undermining democracy."

"We are missing the World Social Forum or something like it at this moment to bring many of the alternatives together, to feel strong and to put our weight on the balance," says Coumba Touré.

An online WSF meeting in June featured "presentations by many people from different organizations across the world, organizations basically of younger people and of people with no previous history with the Social Forum," Edgardo Lander reports. "They saw the WSF as a great possibility." Other examples of new online organizing include a convening in June by the Poor People's Campaign, under the banner of digital justice, and a Global Assembly of the Amazon the following month involving hundreds of organizations and activists from around the world to address the crisis in the Amazon and its inhabitants.

"We need new tools to engage members," Cathy Feingold agrees. "The labor movement is based on old-school face-to-face contact: knocking on doors, holding union meetings in a union hall. So, we're training people on Zoom 101, on how to hold a democratic vote over Zoom, on how to get our brothers and sisters onto the Internet. We are using worker-created organizing apps to engage and mobilize workers. We're teaching leadership how to use this new technology because we may not be face-to-face for a long time."

But activists have to be mindful of the divide between the Internet haves and have-nots. "Distance education undoubtedly increases the already huge distances between the education of the well off and the lower echelons of society worldwide," Edgardo Lander cautions. "What will be the impact on political debate and action of increasing the divide between those who have access to regular, trustworthy Internet service and those who don't?"

The Internet is not just a powerful organizing tool in the hands of progressives. It's also a powerful surveillance tool in the hands of corporations and the government. Indeed, it's part of a new economic form: surveillance capitalism. "I'm not sure our movement completely understands this new form of capitalism," Cathy Feingold worries. "What is our critique of surveillance capitalism and how do we build around it?"

"The very idea of privacy is becoming outdated, privacy in the sense that conversations and exchanges between individuals can be kept away from the eyes and ears of corporations and governments," Edgardo Lander concludes. "What is the possibility of freely debating alternatives, even far-fetched ideas, without risk of being prosecuted as a terrorist? Will this lead to different degrees of self-censorship in political discussions or strategic and tactical debates and planning? This is a major cultural transformation that's been highlighted and accelerated by the present virus situation."

Across Silos

Civil society organizations collaborate across borders largely according to their particular issues—environment, migration, peace. This bureaucratically sensible organizing by silo also allows for more efficient coordination with corresponding international agencies in the UN system. However, it also creates tunnel vision.

A different kind of civil society organizing emerged in the 1990s. "There was global organizing around horrible trade agreements and against the World Bank and IMF," remembers John Cavanagh. "I feel that in the last decade it got more sectoral. A lot of the last decade was the climate movement doing its thing and a lot of creative organizing in the feminist movement. In the United States, we had Occupy, #BlackLivesMatter, Standing Rock, #MeToo. There was great global stuff going on in each of them, but again, sectoral. Presenting a big, sexy alternative to both right-wing fascists and the liberal establishment? We're weaker doing that the stronger we are in our lanes."

The World Social Forum provided an opportunity for movements and organizations to transcend not only national boundaries but issue boundaries as well. But the WSF, too, began to focus in recent years on sectoral issues like extraction and migration. "The WSF played its role, and I think we need something new," Cindy Wiesner says. "Our mistake, particularly in the US and Western concepts of plurality, has been to bring everyone together but at the lowest common denominator. That's the biggest challenge we have in front of us. We have to bring people together with a purpose and a shared outcome. We can't water things down. We need something broader, transformative, and visionary."

The pandemic does offer some opportunities to link issues, such as health care and budget priorities or supply chains and environmental sustainability. "The interwoven crises that we're dealing with—systemic racial and gender inequality, economic inequality, the health crisis, attacks on democracy, and closing space for civil society—these crises are intersectional and connected," notes Cathy Feingold. "We're seeing an amazing moment of cross-movement building. Look at what's happening in Hong Kong and the interconnectedness of their fight for democracy, their fight for justice, and collective action. Here in the United States, climate folks are talking about police reform. The labor movement has links to climate, to gender. How do we sustain cross-sectional movement building over the long term?"

Bringing all of the issues into a single framework, Cindy Wiesner proposes "a just transition to a regenerative, antiracist, feminist economy." The pandemic adds an element of physicality to the equation. "Our physical bodies are the site of the public health crisis," she adds, "but also Black and Brown bodies in particular in relationship to police and state terror. One of the components of that just transition is thinking about bodily autonomy and self-determination, not only your own individual self-determination but self-determination for you as a people."

Targets and Leadership

Much progressive work focuses on the nation-state: electing national leaders, shaping national policy, influencing national debates. Also, there's been a tendency to look to particular nation-states to lead the way in the international arena. Brazil under Luiz Inácio Lula da Silva in the 2000s, for instance, became a progressive beacon in the Global South, forging cooperation among the BRICS nations (Brazil, Russia, India, China, South Africa) as well as providing ideological and financial support to the World Social Forum.

"In the early 2000s, we looked to governments in Bolivia, Ecuador, Venezuela," recalls John Cavanagh. "There's more wariness around that now. But I'm curious what will emerge from South Korea, which held a big election during the pandemic that gave the progressive party a big parliamentary majority on a Green New Deal platform."

The locus of action against the pandemic has been at the national level or lower. True, there have been efforts to forge regional responses, as with the Ecosocial Pact of the South in Latin America and the Caribbean or the work of Africans Rising.[219] But the pandemic has more often redirected attention to the immediate, the urgent, the local. "The more we're impacted globally by this pandemic and these crises, the more our work is going to be hyperlocal and federated regionally," notes Cindy Wiesner. "Speaking as someone who does national and international work, this questions our role as a national alliance."

"The climate organization 350.org is linked with a network of forty cities doing good things on climate," John Cavanagh adds. "A lot of city governments are quite progressive, and they're also getting together globally."

Yet, international institutions have not gone into hibernation during the pandemic. "I get concerned that progressive forces are playing peekaboo: if we don't talk about the IMF, then it's not there," says David Adler. "I'm unnerved by the prospect that, in the rightful resurgence of attention to local ecosystems and communities, we forget that there are powerful institutions pre-shaping those outcomes. At Progressive International, we're working hard to marry local forms of activism to international forms, for instance in campaigns targeting Amazon. We have to match the scale of the activism to the scale of the crisis.

"I say this as a twenty-seven-year-old, medium-proud millennial," he continues. "There's a frustration in my generation about how civil society is vacuum-sealed from politics and economy. When I talk to my team under thirty-five, they find that internationalism comes naturally in way that it may not to their political representatives."

The international labor movement, meanwhile, is operating at all levels. It is pushing on a state-by-state basis for new COVID-19 health standards in the US workplace. At the same time, it's lobbying for a fundamental labor rights standard at the International Labor Organization and pushing for a Global Social Protection Fund at the G20 finance meeting.[220] "If you're going to rebuild resilience, you have to build social protection systems inclusive of everyone," says Cathy Feingold. "It doesn't matter if you're an Ethiopian domestic worker in Saudi Arabia, you should have health care, paid leave, and wage protection when a moment like this hits."

"What are the targets for action that can unite us across silos?" John Cavanagh asks. "The World Bank and International Monetary Fund remain interesting targets. The World Trade Organization is on life support. The World Economic Forum knows that its model is in trouble. The theme of its next meeting is the 'great reset.' It's linking up with Prince Charles, bringing in youth, inviting one of the co-founders of Black Lives Matter, Opal Tometi. They're scrambling for legitimacy. Do we protest outside? Do we have people inside? What are the spaces where we can link together at a moment when the status quo is colossally failing?"

Some of the movements that have emerged in recent years have been essentially leaderless, like the Occupy movement. But examined more closely, even loose networks like the movement for Black Lives Matter have key people who get the ball rolling, invest time and energy over years and sometimes decades, and help determine targets and set priorities.

"There's been a lack of investment into future movement architects," laments Cindy Wiesner. "We have to think of the next society, how the alternatives of, for example, the feminist economy, *buen vivir*, and the commons are in contradiction or complementarity with each other. But we need more focus on the architects, the people on the ground practicing those alternatives, sometimes small in scale, that give us an idea of what can be possible. The current challenge to white supremacy and patriarchy requires new, radical, internationalist, feminist, anti-racist leadership.[221]

"Bringing coherence to movements is our biggest task," she continues. "Some people and movements have seen it as their strategic objective to be weavers and quilters of movements. Just like women's reproductive labor in society, this work is invisible labor that is often marginalized and under-resourced. We have a very transactional model of building coalitions: it's often campaign-based, short-term, 'what can you do for me?' We don't have the basis for coming together around a common frame, values, strategy, vision."

Internationalism

The populist Far Right has attacked institutions of global governance for impinging on the authority of governments to do whatever they want within the boundaries of the nation-state. Leaders like Trump and Bolsonaro have challenged international treaties, global institutions like the World Health Organization, and "globalists" from financiers to human rights campaigners. These right-wing leaders—including Narendra Modi in India, Vladimir Putin in Russia, and Boris Johnson in the UK—have compiled the worst records of dealing with COVID-19.

The institutions of liberal internationalism have also been largely ineffectual during the pandemic. "There's a deep institutional decay in global governance and multilateralism," observes David Adler. "The UN has been notably absent as a forum for international engagement during the pandemic. The WHO is falling apart. The World Bank has followed up on its Washington consensus, with its successor the Wall Street consensus, which is doubling down under its president, David Malpass. This is a high decadent period for these international institutions, which show no signs of being more accountable than in the 1990s."

"A lot of these global institutions are trying to reform or tweak their policies," Cathy Feingold reports. "At the same time, there's the question of whether they're fit for this moment. And we believe that they're really not."

In Europe, David Adler continues, "people like French president Emmanuel Macron are speaking on behalf of a new multilateral energy. But it's a much more ad hoc form of multilateralism, much more constrained and institutionally bound. More disorder will be coming out of this pandemic. We'll be left with leaders who promise the quick fix and don't address the underlying trends like the erosion of the right to health care and the failure to provide basic social goods. This failure to address underlying causes will deliver fresh votes to the Far Right."

If that happens, it would be a replay of the aftermath of the global financial crisis in 2008–9. At that time, remembers Leo Baunach, "a lot of people were thinking that the global financial system is on the backheel, that something new will arise. Ultimately, corporate capture of power was reinforced, and a wave of austerity left people behind. This enabled xenophobic authoritarians to rise to power. We can't count on this being a transformative moment without coordinated strategy."

The World Social Forum represented a different kind of internationalism, a multilateralism from below. "There's been a debate for some time about whether the WSF is still a useful instrument or whether it's no longer seen by the younger generation as the way to go," notes Edgardo Lander. "Let's not kill the Forum. A lot of people think that this meeting of diversities in terms of gender, cultures, and geographic differences has been probably the richest experience we've ever had. Perhaps until we create better alternatives, it would be worthwhile to preserve some form of the WSF, although it is not likely to recover its centrality or its previous scale and transformative energy."

The issue of work can be a unifying global issue during a pandemic, as activists challenge the concept of a "disposable" workforce and go for immediate wins in the realm of health and safety. "It is an interesting opportunity globally to demand that, as people go back to work, we rethink work," John Cavanagh proposes. "Part of that is health and safety and part of that is a democratic debate in which workers are at the center of redefining what health and safety is."

Identity politics, which is often pigeonholed as a form of particularism, "can actually be an opportunity for internationalism," Coumba Touré points out. "If we look at the issue of race, the movement for Black Lives Matter is not only for the United States. It is sparking internationalism by pointing to racism as an ideology that is also the backbone of capitalism, from slavery to colonialism to today's trade relationships. Instead of seeing the feminist movement as something separate, this too is a place of internationalism. It doesn't matter where you are in the world, if you are Black, if you are a woman, if you don't fit the heterosexual norm, you can help the internationalist fight through your identity."

The pandemic is an international crisis, but it has also revealed a crisis in internationalism. "We have reached the limit of the planet," Edgardo Lander points out. "There's a need to think and act in terms of the possibility of another civilization, of going beyond the debate on state and market. We need to go beyond the logic of this industrial society, this individualistic, possessive conception of the human being. These possibilities are opened up by this sense of a shared experience of the pandemic."

Chapter 7: International Civil Society Discussion Participants

DAVID ADLER is a political economist whose work focuses on the politics of internationalism: how social movements coordinate across borders, and how international institutions aid or impede those efforts. He is the coordinator for the Progressive International movement. Currently based in Florence, Italy, he's a policy leader fellow at the School of Transnational Governance at the European University Institute. He also serves as the policy director for the Democracy in Europe Movement 2025 (DiEM25) and the coordinator of its Green New Deal for Europe campaign. His writing has appeared in the *New York Times*, the *Guardian*, and *Boston Review*.

LEO BAUNACH is the director of the International Trade Union Confederation and Global Unions Office in Washington, DC, which advocates for reforming multilateralism and a development model that benefits working people everywhere.

JOHN CAVANAGH has been director of the Institute for Policy Studies (IPS) in Washington, DC, since 1999. He directed IPS's Global Economy Program from 1983 to 1997. He is the co-author of twelve books and numerous articles on a wide range of social and economic issues. He sits on the boards of the Congressional Progressive Caucus Center, the International Forum on Globalization, International Labor Rights Forum, the Fund for Constitutional Government, and the New Economy Coalition. He worked as an economist for the United Nations Conference on Trade and Development (1978–81) and the World Health Organization (1981–82). He served on the Civil Society Advisory Committee of the UN Development Program (2000–12).

CATHY FEINGOLD is the director of the AFL-CIO's International Department in Washington, DC. In 2018, she was elected deputy president of the International Trade Union Confederation, the organization representing two hundred million unionized workers worldwide. She previously directed the AFL-CIO Solidarity Center's work in the Dominican Republic and Haiti, where she worked with local trade union partners to develop innovative campaigns to improve the working conditions of domestic, migrant, and informal economy workers. Her professional experience includes work for the labor movement, large international organizations, small grassroots NGOs, and a foundation. She has written about the impact of economic policies on market women in Nigeria, and, as a Fulbright Scholar in Nicaragua, she researched the impact of structural adjustment policies on women workers.

EDGARDO LANDER is professor emeritus of sociology at the Central University of Venezuela, a professor at the Universidad Indígena de Venezuela and at the Universidad Andina Simón Bolívar in Quito, a permanent member of the Global Working Group Beyond Development, and one of the organizers of the 2006 World Social Forum in Caracas. In 2017, Edgardo was a founding member of the Plataforma Ciudadana en Defensa de la Constitución (Citizen Platform in Defense of the Constitution) comprised of former Chavistas, who became highly critical of his successor. Edgardo is the author of numerous books and research articles on the environmental limits to industrialization and economic growth, the Left in government in Latin America, post-democratic capitalism, and challenges to Eurocentric epistemologies.

COUMBA TOURÉ, a writer and storyteller, was born and raised between Mali and Senegal. She is the co-coordinator of Africans Rising for Justice, Peace and Dignity and a board member of TrustAfrica. She publishes children's stories and organizes art events targeting children's minds through Falia. She also designs popular education programs with a focus to impact women and children. She has extensive experience in facilitating meetings internationally, engaging young people, designing, implementing, and evaluating training programs to promote human rights, especially those of women. Coumba has promoted social entrepreneurship through her work with Ashoka for the past ten years. She has worked with organizations such as the Institute for Popular Education in Mali, the 21st Century Youth Leadership Movement in Selma, Alabama, and the Youth for Environmental Sanity in Santa Cruz, California. She is a member of the African Feminist Forum and the Per Ankh collective.

CINDY WIESNER is the executive director of Grassroots Global Justice Alliance, based in Florida. A twenty-five-year veteran of the social justice movement in the United States and internationally, she helped co-found the Climate Justice Alliance and has played a leadership role in the Peoples Climate Movement that organized the massive mobilizations in New York, Washington, DC, and San Francisco in recent years, and is an adviser to Groundswell's Liberation Fund. She started organizing with HERE Local 2850 in Oakland, California, and went on to become the director of organizing for People Organizing to Win Employment Rights in San Francisco and an organizer and board member for generationFIVE. She has also been a consultant for Men Overcoming Violence Everywhere and Mujeres Unidas y Activas. She previously worked as leadership development director of the Miami Workers Center and represented the group as a member of the US Social Forum National Planning Committee. She has been active in many movement building initiatives over the years, including World March of Women, Social Movement Assemblies, International Council of the World Social Forum, Fight Against the FTAA, UNITY, Building Equity and Alignment Initiative, and, currently, It Takes Roots and the Rising Majority.

CHAPTER 8:
INTERNATIONAL COOPERATION

In 2003, the international community faced a new type of epidemic: severe acute respiratory syndrome. SARS would eventually spread to more than thirty countries, infecting about eight thousand people and killing around eight hundred. This mortality rate of 10 percent would have produced a catastrophic death toll if SARS had surged in the general population.

It took six months to beat back the SARS epidemic, thanks in large part to the World Health Organization (WHO). According to a US team of researchers, "The central role of WHO in coordinating the laboratory network that identified the etiologic agent and shared reagents, the epidemiology network that characterized the spread and identified the most effective control measures, and the policy and communications network that incorporated rapidly changing knowledge into measured travel advisories was critical for the control of the epidemic and a credit to WHO."[222]

In the wake of SARS, the WHO also came up with new guidelines for responding to future outbreaks. These regulations were legally binding, and 196 countries signed the framework agreement. But ten years later, only 20 percent of the signatories had implemented the core requirements.[223]

It was hardly a surprise, when COVID-19 hit in 2020, that all of this patient international cooperation unraveled. Dozens of countries, as Selam Gebrekidan reported in the *New York Times* in March, "are flouting the international regulations and snubbing their obligations. Some have failed to report outbreaks to the organization, as required. Others have instituted international travel restrictions, against the advice of the WHO, and without notifying global health officials."[224]

Compared to the international success in combatting SARS in 2003, the obvious international failure to contain COVID-19 in 2020 says much about the nature of global cooperation in an age of surging nationalism. To cite but one difference, the United States fully cooperated with the WHO in 2003. By 2020, although US experts participated in the early WHO meetings about the new disease in Wuhan, the United States announced its intention in July to withdraw from the organization.

"The decline of the European Union, the withdrawal of the United States from the WHO and other international institutions, the overall deterioration of the international system of working together: How much has the COVID emergency pushed countries to turn inward instead of seeking to cooperate?" asks Diana Ohlbaum of the Friends Committee on National Legislation.

The retreat of the United States behind geopolitical walls, tariff walls, and literal walls has not only been a major part of this turn inward, it has also altered the global power balance.

"The shift toward a lopsided multipolarity is accelerating," says Rachel Esplin Odell of the Quincy Institute. "In the United States, in particular, there's a sense that we're shifting away from a unipolar world."

China, too, has contributed to this lopsided multipolarity. Although it was the first country to face COVID-19, China was also the first to control the virus. Even as much of the world continues to suffer economically from lockdown policies, the Chinese economy quickly rebounded with significant growth after a first-quarter contraction of nearly 7 percent.[225] China is emerging from the pandemic in a stronger global position than, say, the United States or Russia.

But the pandemic has also sharpened conflict between Beijing and Washington, with both sides trading charges of complicity in the spread of COVID-19. This deepening animosity comes at a particularly inopportune time. "The Trump administration is overreaching in ways that are obvious to many people who think that international cooperation around pandemic management with China is essential regardless of what you think about China's behavior in Hong Kong and Xinjiang," argues Richard Javad Heydarian, an Asia-based academic and columnist.

The United Nations, meanwhile, has been noticeably absent from a pandemic response, at least at the highest levels. The secretary general called for a global ceasefire in March that largely went unheeded. "At the global level, particularly in the UN, it's a mess: the member states can't even agree to a least common denominator," explains Jens Martens of the Global Policy Forum. "At a high-level forum on sustainable development, they couldn't reach any agreement, not even a statement of jargon. At the official UN level, there's no way to reach any agreement with the Trump administration and many others."

Meanwhile, as governments shut down international travel and key links in global supply chains, the pandemic has disrupted the circulatory system of economic globalization. "The pandemic is reconfiguring globalization and in particular global value chains," observes Fiona Dove of the Transnational Institute. "Will we see more focus on regional economies or more of an attempt to diversify supply chains? Either way, I don't think we're going back to the way it was."

The pandemic has had differential impact across countries and within countries. "It's not true that we're all in the same boat," points out Tobita Chow of Justice Is Global. "Even so, our destinies are connected. We need international cooperation to beat this thing and, further, to develop solutions. None of us will be safe until all of us are safe. This was already true, but the pandemic makes that clearer than ever."

Multipolarity

After the end of the Cold War, the United States presided over a unipolar world. The Soviet Union was gone, Russia was weak, China was still playing catch-up, and Europe was focused on internal consolidation. But despite its preponderant military and economic power, the United States could not dictate outcomes on the ground, failing in the 1990s to stop the genocide in Rwanda and the ethnic cleansing in Yugoslavia. In the 2000s, with America focused on regime change in Afghanistan and the greater Middle East, a new multipolar world emerged: the "rise of the rest."[226] China surged to superpower status on the strength of its annual double-digit economic growth and military budget increases. Middle powers like Brazil and India rose to greater prominence. Russia managed to regain a measure of the Soviet Union's global status.

The pandemic, in accentuating America's relative decline of power in the world, has encouraged this long-term trend toward multipolarity. "The vacuum of leadership provided by the Trump administration over the last three years has nudged other countries to step up to the plate: Europe, Japan, South Korea, Indonesia," observes Richard Javad Heydarian. "Even if Joe Biden wins the US presidential election, we won't go back to the status quo ante of America leading the world. It will be a more coherent and cooperative America dealing with more competent, proactive middle powers, which have gradually embraced a post-American world. This is a more ideal outcome than just leaving the world to China or returning to the liberal hegemony of the Clinton-to-Obama era."

"Multipolarity, as I understand it, increases the threat of war, including trade war," observes Samuel Moyn of Yale University. "But it seems that the default view among progressives is that more multipolarity is a good thing. The challenge is how to manage it: avoiding the risks while coaxing the opportunities."

"Multipolarity is a good thing in that it imposes constraints on the excesses of great powers in particular," agrees Rachel Esplin Odell. "Multipolarism requires countries to be more judicious in their use of power."

Richard Javad Heydarian, however, is not so sure. "In progressive circles, we take it as an article of faith that multipolarity is always good," he notes. "But if you're the Philippines, Ukraine, or Bahrain, countries on the geopolitical front line, multipolarity means that China will dominate East Asia, Iran will dominate the Persian Gulf, and Russia will dominate the post-Soviet space. Maybe multipolarity means less American hyperpower domination, but the actual impact on the ground could be—and is perceived as—different."

The pandemic has also introduced a dismal alternative to a multipolar or unipolar order: no order whatsoever. In response to the last major economic crisis in 2008–9, "we saw G20 coordination happening at the highest possible level, with Angela Merkel in Germany and Barack Obama getting their acts together," Heydarian remembers. "Now where's the leader? This is an absolute case of apolarity. The Chinese and Americans are shouting at each other in international fora. The Europeans and Japanese are trying their best to squeeze themselves in. The rest of us in the post-colonial world are wondering where the help will come from. We don't want to be left with private corporations for the future of our vaccines and our public health."

It's not only the post-colonial world that has taken note of the absence of international coordination during this pandemic. "There's a lot of idealistic thinking that, in a crisis, people come together," observes Diana Ohlbaum. "But almost the opposite has happened right from the start, with recriminations over who's at fault, countries competing for supplies and equipment, and companies competing to develop a vaccine. In this crisis, we have defaulted to competition and violence rather than cooperation and peacemaking."[227]

Accompanying this decline in international cooperation has been increased militarism. "The clash between China and India, Israel maybe attacking Iran, increasing tensions between the United States and China: we're in the middle of a pandemic crisis plus an economic crisis, but some people are trying do their best to add a crisis of militarism," concludes Tobita Chow.

US-China Stand-Off

As the pandemic gathered force in the United States, the Trump administration increasingly blamed China for the outbreak as it applied a series of sanctions: over Beijing's crackdown on dissent in Hong Kong, against Chinese social media platforms TikTok and WeChat, in response to the treatment of the Uighur minority.[228] The United States closed the Chinese consulate in Houston, made high-level complaints about Chinese actions in the South China Sea, and continued to draw together allies from India to Australia into an Indo-Pacific alliance against China.[229] In a speech in July, Secretary of State Mike Pompeo effectively declared the end of engagement with China and a shift toward supporting regime change.[230] The Pentagon tightened its policy of military containment.[231]

China has responded in kind to many of the US actions by imposing sanctions on a number of Americans, including senators Marco Rubio (F-FL) and Ted Cruz (R-TX), and closing the US consulate in Chengdu. "The rise of anti-China sentiment in United States has been matched in China," notes Tobita Chow. "There have been a lot of anti-US narratives, including a popular conspiracy theory that the US military introduced the pandemic into Wuhan."

China has also become more assertive in its neighborhood. "Over the last three months, we've seen brazen Chinese strategic opportunism and revanchism in the South China Sea," reports Richard Javad Heydarian. "When the United States got bogged down with the USS *Roosevelt* pandemic outbreak and it became impossible for countries in this region to do joint exercises, the Chinese made the most of it and continued to build facts on the ground, in contravention of international law and the interests of smaller nations."[232]

"The tensions that have taken place this year, including China's sinking of a Vietnamese fishing boat in April, are not new but have precedent in previous years," Rachel Esplin Odell points out. "Thus, they probably don't have much to do with the pandemic. Moreover, the disputes in the South China Sea are about more than just China against the rest. They are highly complex and multisided. There is an urgent need for China and the other states around the South China Sea to work together on a more cooperative basis to manage disputes around resource extraction and conservation, rather than allowing these disputes to escalate into conflict."

Some countries, like Australia, have pursued a tougher policy toward China during the pandemic. But, Odell continues, "there's a growing disconnect between how the United States sees its relationship with China and China's role in the world, and the way the rest of the world views it. The United States increasingly sees the relationship in Manichean terms, pursuing a bipolar cold war–style competition. Most of the rest of the world views China as a major power that's necessary to get along with in order to solve international problems."

This more hostile approach may backfire by strengthening Chinese leader Xi Jinping's legitimacy at home. "Increasing conflict with the United States builds popular nationalist sentiment, which translates into support for the regime," explains Tobita Chow. "And the fact that China's response to the pandemic has been effective, compared to the incompetent US response, is a source of national pride."

Countries in China's vicinity might see things differently. Taiwan and South Korea both successfully handled the pandemic—and without the kind of lockdown that China imposed. "No one believes that the COVID-19 numbers in China are anywhere close to reality," says Richard Javad Heydarian. "According to one survey, seventy-five percent of Filipinos want accountability. Australia has turned against China in ways that were unthinkable a year or two ago. Xi will use popular nationalism and xenophobia as a fallback option. But that is going to have a cost."

The cold war into which the US-China relationship is descending differs fundamentally from the Cold War that dominated the second half of the last century. The United States and the Soviet Union never had much of an economic relationship. By contrast, the economies of the United States and China have become mutually dependent.

But the Trump administration is working to change that. "For a long time, the ballast in the US-China relationship has rested in the economic sector, in the incentives that states have to compete for Chinese investment or export opportunities," Rachel Esplin Odell observes. "The Trump administration proactively targeted those industries. Pompeo gave a speech before the pandemic to governors warning them against cooperation with China. In July, FBI director Christopher Wray gave a similar speech to companies warning of their becoming unwitting Chinese agents."

This anti-China strategy also has an electoral component. "The US Right, the Republican Party, the Trump administration: they see anti-Chinese politics as their key to reelection," notes Tobita Chow. "Despite the rise of anti-Chinese sentiment in the United States, polling shows that if you ask people to choose between cooperation with China to beat the pandemic versus confronting China or holding China accountable, a strong majority of people prefer international cooperation."[233]

Rachel Esplin Odell agrees that the "dramatic downturn in the relationship has outpaced the domestic US support that exists for it. It has also provoked some Democrats and people on the left to realize that this slide toward confrontation with China has gone too far. Hopefully there can be some pulling away from geopolitical confrontation if the US election goes as polls indicate. There are grounds for optimism that the logic and narrative of common-sense cooperation around shared interests can be extended to climate change and cutting the defense budget, although unfortunately Congress hasn't caught up with that."

Progressives have to develop a nuanced approach to the challenge of China, Richard Javad Heydarian argues. "There's a lot of criticism of Trump's approach, but there are also some legitimate and disturbing concerns about the rise of China," he maintains. "We have to find an approach that preserves the sovereignty of smaller countries around China who feel that their sovereignty is threatened in digital and maritime disputes. We have to dispense with the idea that any challenge to the United States is automatically a good thing. It matters who is the challenger and what it stands for. A lot of people in the region would rather have a liberal hegemon than an illiberal hegemon like China. But, as a progressive, I believe it should be about transcending both superpowers."

Multilateralism and the UN

The United Nations has not played a critical role during COVID-19—at least not in the Security Council or General Assembly. But international cooperation has prospered elsewhere in the UN system.

"The WHO just created an independent panel for pandemic preparedness and response," reports Jens Martens. "The presidents of Canada and Jamaica launched a new initiative at the UN level on financing for development in the COVID-19 era and beyond. A new Financial Accountability, Transparency and Integrity panel is looking at illicit financial flows. There's a lot of new multilateral action just below the General Assembly by those who don't want to wait for it to reach consensus. Perhaps this is a second-best solution as long as we have Trump, Bolsonaro, Duterte, and all the others."[234]

"The rise of right-wing populist nationalism predated the pandemic," Rachel Esplin Odell points out. "It's possible that there will be a lag time before the pandemic has a political cost for those actors. Once it does, and if we see a shift to a Joe Biden administration in the United States, the trend away from multilateralism might reverse."

In the meantime, the pandemic is encouraging a transformation of multilateralism toward public-private initiatives. The most recent example is the effort by Gavi, the Vaccine Alliance, to fund the acquisition of vaccines in countries.

"The United States, the United Kingdom, and the United Nations are appealing to other states and the public to fund this privately run effort to decide the allocation of vaccines when they're available by purchasing them in a commercial market and then testing this vaccine in developing countries," explains Harris Gleckman of the Center for Governance and Sustainability at the University of Massachusetts Boston.

The reconfiguration of multilateralism in the direction of global partnerships between the public and private sectors has developed over the course of three decades. "This trend toward multistakeholderism is now strengthened during the COVID-19 pandemic," explains Jens Martens. "The World Economic Forum (WEF) is trying to position itself in the center of the response with its 'Great Reset' summit in 2021 in Davos and with hundreds of subconferences all over planet. The 'great reset' means: start capitalism from the beginning because it doesn't work now." Still, inter-governmental institutions like the World Bank and International Monetary Fund want to be at the center of the recovery, and the private sector certainly doesn't want to go it alone. "Even corporate activists and lobbyists are now calling for more governmental and inter-governmental action," he adds.

A major problem with global governance is the voluntary nature of compliance. The Paris climate agreement, for instance, established certain benchmarks by which countries reduce their carbon emissions, but those goals were entirely voluntary. "Voluntarism sounds great, it's what you do in your neighborhood," Harris Gleckman points out. "But what it means is: let the powerful do what they want when they want to do it, and if they don't there's no consequence. According to the WEF view of the world, we can't force anyone to do anything, even if it's inherently bad for billions of people and the environment."

Arms control agreements, with their verification protocols, are a better model. But these agreements haven't fared well either in the age of right-wing populism. Under Trump, the United States unsigned the Arms Trade Treaty, which went into effect in 2014. Trump pulled out of the Open Skies agreement, signed in 1992, and the Intermediate-Range Nuclear Forces treaty, signed in 1987. And he trashed the Iran nuclear agreement. Instead of pursuing denuclearization, as mandated by the Nuclear Non-Proliferation Treaty, the nuclear club members are all modernizing their forces, at great cost.[235] The UN helplessly watches the unravelling of the arms-control system.

Nor has the UN been able to do much about the unravelling of the global economy. The United Nations was established in 1945 largely to prevent another world war from taking place. The Bretton Woods system of the IMF and World Bank, created the year before, was intended to prevent another Great Depression. "We may have to think about a multilateralism that has another major branch to govern globalization," Harris Gleckman continues. "Over the last twenty years, under the push for the deregulation of the state, delegates have stepped back even further from attempting to govern globalization. But globalization is a vulnerability. We have an old system but new types of crises."

Globalization

After the pandemic first hit, the global economy shuddered when China closed its factories. Economic shutdowns followed in one country after another, and the circulatory system of global trade suffered a series of paralyzing strokes.

"We've seen a catastrophic failure of the global free market with competition over medical supplies, hoarding and price gouging, governments stealing masks from each other," says Tobita Chow. "This reveals a need for countries to come together in an alternative system that's more rational and meets actual human needs like greater investment globally into health infrastructure and international cooperation around developing a people's vaccine."

The breakdown of supply chains during the pandemic not only bankrupted businesses and distressed consumers, it threw millions of people out of work. One group of affected workers that has not received much attention are the seafarers who run container vessels and cruise ships. "The Philippines has the second-largest number of seafarers after China," explains Richard Javad Heydarian. "A lot of them are stuck and can't go home. A growing number of them have committed suicide. The governments of the Philippines, Indonesia, and India earned tens of billions of dollars from seafarers and overseas workers. Shame on them for not creating a mechanism to expedite their return."[236]

Right-wing populists like Trump and Hungarian prime minister Viktor Orbán are opposed not just to the "globalists" installed in the UN bureaucracy. They have criticized the investors and financiers who participate in economic globalization. "The dominant strain of nationalism influences how people think of supply chains," notes Tobita Chow. "In the United States, the key phrase in localizing supply chains is 'national security.' Preferable would be more resilient supply chains based on international cooperation rather than a fear of foreign threats."

The pandemic marks a time when "we should bring back the traditional left obsession with class and work both within nations and in the supply chains across nations," suggests Samuel Moyn. This focus should encompass those who expose themselves to infection by merely showing up to work.

The International Labor Organization (ILO) has put out regular updates on COVID-19 and the world of work, with estimates of the loss of working hours, the disproportionate impact of the shutdowns on women workers, and recommendations for a job-rich recovery.[237] The ILO has also received attention for its study of the increasing impact of artificial intelligence on the workplace, which the pandemic is accelerating.[238] "The Asian Development Bank study in 2018 said, 'Don't worry, whatever job goes away there will be new jobs,'" reports Richard Javad Heydarian. "It was the usual technophilia. But the ILO showed that a lot of low-skilled workers will lose their jobs. And even if they keep their jobs, it will be the worst version of the precariat."[239]

Tech companies have largely prospered during the pandemic. In the first full quarter of COVID-19, although the US economy contracted by 32 percent, the big four (Apple, Amazon, Facebook, Google) took in nearly $30 billion in profits.[240] "The big tech companies are moving in and moving fast" to translate their market position into political power, notes Fiona Dove. "The tech companies are very active in the World Economic Forum space as well."

Globally, the well-off have managed to weather the economic shutdowns. By the end of summer 2020, the stock markets had largely recovered the value they lost when the pandemic hit. Instead of forming a V shape, the recovery looks more like a K, with a sharp divergence in the fortunes of rich and poor.[241] "Asset inequality is going to happen much faster," Harris Gleckman predicts. "The central bank chose to underwrite the stock market and those investors in dramatic fashion. The Federal Reserve will put an estimated ten trillion dollars toward supporting bonds, stocks, and other financial instruments. That's roughly half the GDP of the United States."

Over the summer of 2020, the European Union wrestled with this issue of equitable outcomes coming out of the pandemic. "There's a big fight about solidarity," Fiona Dove reports. "Europe is basically run by accountants: there's not much politics. The fight is over the rate of interest of loan repayment for Italy, which is in danger of collapse altogether, threatening the future of the monetary union." In the ultimate compromise, Italy and other heavily indebted members received about half of the $858 billion EU bailout assistance in the form of grants.[242]

Role of the State

The pandemic has served as a ruthless test of a state's competence. Its impact varies widely, from countries with only a handful of deaths like Vietnam, Thailand, New Zealand, and Uruguay to places overwhelmed by sickness and death like the United Kingdom and Peru. The four countries with the worst record of managing COVID-19—the United States, Brazil, India, and Russia—also happen to be led by right-wing nationalists.

"Once again we're seeing that disaster in general, and public health in particular, are crucial sources of legitimation of political authority," observes Samuel Moyn. "States and international institutions suffer badly when they fail in this realm. In the United States, George W. Bush got hurt far less by Iraq than by Hurricane Katrina. We're seeing Trump felled by, of all the terrible things he's done, his handling of this disease."

"With the notable exception of Viktor Orbán, who loves to shut down borders, the populists are not doing well," notes Richard Javad Heydarian. "Their incompetence has been exposed like never before. Yet, they're using the opportunity of the pandemic, namely the difficulty of protest and normal civil disobedience campaigns, to consolidate power and isolate the opposition in preemptive ways. Here, in the Philippines, the government closed the largest TV network, jailed journalists, and passed a new anti-terror law. This government is busy with everything except dealing with the virus. If there's any silver lining in this, we're also seeing the rise of post-populists, a new generation of young progressive mayors. They have the populist charisma, they're very good on social media, they're young, but they use their charisma to push for progressive values."[243]

The issue of competence will have implications beyond the pandemic. "Increasingly, domestic capacity as opposed to military power is going to be seen as a source of national power," observes Rachel Esplin Odell. "Those countries with dysfunctional political systems or insufficient state capacity will come out of this crisis further weakened. It's unrelated to regime type. Whether authoritarian or democratic, those countries with more state capacity for crisis response or public health are faring better."

"We see that clearly in the Philippines," Richard Javad

Heydarian agrees. "The economy has been growing very fast, six to seven percent a year. The government has easy access to billions of dollars in loans from multilateral agencies to deal with the crisis. And yet, four months into the pandemic, these guys haven't been able to put together a detailed stimulus program. It's the sheer incompetence and weakness of state institutions to mobilize all the existing resources to deal with the crisis."

Some countries have responded effectively, and "that might enhance trust in the state," Rachel Esplin Odell points out. "We may see that in the case of China. Certainly, there are ways that the government responded that have raised suspicions and weakened its image domestically, and that extends to the continued clampdown on civil liberties in Hong Kong and the disappearing domestically of prominent critics of the government. But obviously they were able to contain the pandemic quite well after the early stages, and this plays into how the Chinese government portrays itself through domestic propaganda efforts. So, they actually might come out stronger domestically, though their behavior has weakened their international standing to some extent."

In the United States, the mishandling of the pandemic has not led to a reevaluation of the country's role in the world or its budget priorities at home. And it's not just the fault of the Trump administration. "The US Congress has its head stuck in the sand," observes Diana Ohlbaum. "There's no big thinking in Congress about a change in US foreign policy or how we redefine national interest. No matter how loud those calls are coming from the outside, they have not made it to Congress at all." One example is the annual authorization of funds for the military, which "will continue at $741 billion as if nothing has changed," she adds.

As the federal government fails, attention turns to other levels of authority. "Of course, we need progressive internationalism," notes Samuel Moyn. "But I wonder if we're learning the lesson that we can work at different scales. What are the prospects for cities and for regions to have foreign policies that do better than nation-states and international institutions?"

Jens Martens is struck by a similar question. "How can we expect a strengthened UN by the same national leaders who fail at the national level?" he asks. "Perhaps we should be looking at multilevel not multistakeholder governance. We should look into the cooperation of cities, for instance, through the global coalition United Cities and Local Governments, which is working together on sustainable development. This is interesting, but I don't see it as an alternative. We should not just focus on cities and get rid of the nation-state, but we should take them more into account and see how they can fill the gaps created by incompetent nationalist leaders at the national level."

"More and more, progressive movements are looking to the city level as a source of hope and also a level that's much more accountable, easier to engage and organize," Fiona Dove adds. "But there are obstacles. The WTO puts obstacles in the way of what cities are able to do to promote local employment or source things locally."

Cities are also leading a trend away from privatization. "There are more than a thousand initiatives, mostly at the local community level, that have led to a remunicipalization of services," Jens Martens points out. "There's also a consensus at the international level that the privatization of health systems was a failure." This consensus, he adds, should shape the disbursement of stimulus funds so that they do not, as in the United States, go largely to vested interests.[244]

Movement Responses

International cooperation has emerged, if only in a dispersed way, in the protests that have rippled across the globe "not only in the last couple months but in the last twelve to twenty-four months," Jens Martens observes. "There were a lot of mass protests all over the world, not related necessarily to COVID response but mainly responding to discrimination and the impact of austerity policies. There were millions of people on the street in Argentina, Lebanon, South Africa, Ecuador, and Egypt. The Black Lives Matter movement reached a global level, like the Fridays for Future and Extinction Rebellion before. What we don't have is a unified movement that deals with multiple crises in a trans-sectoral, interdisciplinary sense."

The pandemic has performed a certain function in this regard. "It has stripped away the obfuscations around who benefits from the way the current system is organized, and that's led to a lot of public anger," reports Diana Ohlbaum.

That public anger can be channeled into positive transformation—or it can, as after the 2008–9 financial crisis, translate into support for right-wing populism. "If we as progressives push for radical change, we have to reassure people that it won't lead to more disorder. Otherwise, it gives ammunition to authoritarian leaders who will say, 'You need me even more because these crazy people will make it worse,'" Richard Javad Heydarian points out. "We have to think about basic safety and basic challenges to existence for people who have nothing to hold onto during this moment of crisis. Will radical rhetoric really attract them? This is a great opportunity for a reset not in a neoliberal but in a progressive sense. But it has to be expressed in language that appeals to average, reasonable people who don't necessarily buy into our worldview."

The pandemic has also highlighted a central tension in organizing—between achieving victories at the international level and winning elections at the national level. "I haven't seen any progressive gurus who have a vision of how to square the national and the supranational without wishing away the potential conflicts between policymaking at different levels," says Samuel Moyn.

"The way progressives have been organizing—stove-piped by issue, with people in the United States who do international development, for instance, talking to those who do similar work in other countries—may need at least temporarily to be converted to organizing across issues *within* countries, leaving international coordination until we get our acts together in our own countries," Diana Ohlbaum notes. "The current structure perpetuates a divide between what we consider 'foreign' and 'domestic' issues, when what we need to do is recognize their interconnections."

"The need for greater international cooperation is so urgent and the threat of growing nationalism is such a present danger that we have to do both at once," urges Tobita Chow. "But how do we articulate an internationalist platform in a way that doesn't seem so radical that we inadvertently feed popular support for authoritarianism?" He points to the example of Hong Kong, where militant protest alienated members of the professional elite and the finance sector that initially supported the demonstrators. Meanwhile, in the United States, he continues, "we need to figure out how to pitch internationalism within a framework of American leadership, because we still have this dominant narrative of American exceptionalism, the idea of the United States as world leader, that's in stark contradiction to international cooperation or any progressive multilateralism."

"It's political suicide to challenge the notion of US global leadership," agrees Diana Ohlbaum. "But we need to show people why that is problematic and offer alternative visions of a constructive US role in the world."

In the meantime, the pandemic shows no sign of disappearing. Even when it does, "we're still looking at a multi-year economic, health, and environmental crisis," Harris Gleckman concludes. "Progressives have to do the big thinking both on how to survive these multi-year crises and how to propose a different frame of reference for the process afterward."

Chapter 8: International Cooperation Discussion Participants

TOBITA CHOW is the director of Justice Is Global, a special project of People's Action to create a more just and sustainable global economy and defeat right-wing nationalism. Based in Chicago, he is organizing a progressive internationalist alternative to the growing tensions between the United States and China.

FIONA DOVE has been executive director of the Transnational Institute in Amsterdam since 1995. She grew up in South Africa, where she was an anti-apartheid activist from a young age, and later served as a national negotiator and research coordinator for the SA Commercial, Catering and Allied Workers' Union. She serves on the board of De Goede Zaak (Netherlands), the Pluto Educational Trust (UK), the advisory board of the Erasmus Mundus Master in Global Studies coordinated by the University of Leipzig, and the editorial advisory board of the journal *Development in Practice*.

HARRIS GLECKMAN is a senior fellow at the Center for Governance and Sustainability at the University of Massachusetts Boston and director of benchmark environmental consulting. He was a staff member of the UN Centre on Transnational Corporations, head of the New York office of the United Nations Conference on Trade and Development, and an early member of the staff for the 2002 Monterey Conference on Financing for Development.

RICHARD HEYDARIAN has taught political science at De La Salle University and Ateneo De Manila University, and is an incoming research fellow at National Chengchi University in Taiwan. He is currently resident analyst at GMA Network, a columnist for the Philippine *Daily Inquirer*, and a regular opinion writer for leading global publications. His latest book is *The Rise of Duterte: A Populist Revolt against Elite Democracy* (Palgrave), and he is also the author of *The IndoPacific Age: Trump, China, and the New Global Struggle for Mastery* (Palgrave), as well as *Duterte's Foreign Policy*. He is a regular contributor to the Council on Foreign Relations and Center for Strategic and International Studies in Washington, DC, and has written for and/or been interviewed by Al Jazeera, BBC, Bloomberg, CNN, the *New York Times*, the *Washington Post*, the *Guardian*, the *Wall Street Journal*, *Foreign Affairs*, *Foreign Policy*, and the *Economist*, among other leading global publications.

JENS MARTENS has been executive director of Global Policy Forum (New York/Bonn) since its founding in 2004. Since 2011, he has coordinated the international Civil Society Reflection Group on the 2030 Agenda for Sustainable Development. From 2003 to 2009, he was member (2006–9 co-chair) of the Coordinating Committee of Social Watch, a global network of several hundred NGOs working on poverty eradication and social justice. Previously, he was a longstanding member of the executive board of the German NGO World Economy, Ecology and Development (WEED). From 1997 until 2004, he worked at WEED as director of its Programs on International Environment and Development Policy and on Corporate Accountability. Prior to joining the staff at WEED, he worked as a freelance author and adviser for several NGOs and foundations, including the German NGO Forum on Environment and Development, the Friedrich Ebert Foundation, and the Development and Peace Foundation. He has published more than one hundred articles in journals, newspapers, and handbooks, has written several books and studies on development policy and UN reform, and has been co-editor of three books on German UN policy, privatization, and corporate accountability.

SAMUEL MOYN is Henry R. Luce Professor of Jurisprudence at Yale Law School and professor of history at Yale University. His areas of interest in legal scholarship include international law, human rights, the law of war, and legal thought, in both historical and current perspective. In intellectual history, he has worked on a diverse range of subjects, especially twentieth-century European moral and political theory. He has written several books in his fields of European intellectual history and human rights history, including *The Last Utopia: Human Rights in History* (2010), and edited or co-edited a number of others. His most recent books are *Christian Human Rights* (2015, based on Mellon Distinguished Lectures at the University of Pennsylvania in fall 2014) and *Not Enough: Human Rights in an Unequal World* (2018). He is currently working on a new book on the origins and significance of humane war for Farrar, Straus and Giroux. Over the years, he has written in venues such as *Boston Review*, the *Chronicle of Higher Education*, *Dissent*, the *Nation*, the *New Republic*, the *New York Times*, and the *Wall Street Journal*.

RACHEL ESPLIN ODELL is a PhD candidate in international relations and comparative politics and a member of the MIT Security Studies Program. She is also an international security fellow at Harvard Kennedy School's Belfer Center for Science and International Affairs and a research fellow at the Quincy Institute for Responsible Statecraft in Washington, DC. Her dissertation explains differences in states' interpretation of the international law of the sea and the evolution in those interpretations over time. Her broader research interests include the nature and future of world order, US strategy in the Asia-Pacific region, Chinese foreign policy, and crisis management in Northeast Asia. She previously worked as a research analyst in the Asia Program at the Carnegie Endowment for International Peace.

DIANA OHLBAUM directs the Friends Committee on National Legislation's (FCNL) foreign policy lobbying team in Washington, DC, and leads an effort to replace the current US foreign policy paradigm of military domination and national superiority with a more ethical and effective one based on cooperation and mutual respect. She brings to FCNL nearly two decades of experience on Capitol Hill, where she served as a senior professional staff member of both the House Foreign Affairs Committee and the Senate Foreign Relations Committee, and earlier as an aide to Senator Paul S. Sarbanes (D-MD). During her time as a congressional staff member, Diana coordinated efforts to overhaul the outdated Foreign Assistance Act of 1961, improve oversight of arms sales and security assistance, and promote diplomacy and multilateralism. From 1999 to 2001, she served as deputy director of USAID's Office of Transition Initiatives, a cutting-edge unit designed to advance peace and democracy in priority conflict-prone countries. She also worked as director of public policy for InterAction, an alliance of NGOs engaged in humanitarian relief and international development.

AN END TO EXCEPTIONALISM?

For days, weeks, and months, the COVID-19 pandemic has forced hundreds of millions of people to shelter in place, maintain "social distance," and limit their contact with others.

In the international arena, too, countries have limited their contacts with others. They have closed borders, restricted travel, and reduced economic and political interaction. Every country has, in a sense, sheltered in place. They have focused on ministering to their own citizens and reviving their own economies.

As this book demonstrates, international cooperation has been in short supply during this pandemic. Countries have competed for scarce medical resources. The race for a vaccine has been national, for the most part, not international. Where neighbors have been in contact—Saudi Arabia and Yemen, India and China, Israel and Syria—more often it has been to make war, not common cause.

The pandemic has encouraged a certain myopia, a national nearsightedness, a failure to see the bigger picture.

Nationalism was already on the rise pre-pandemic. Worse,

the major powers were practicing a dangerous exceptionalism that was eroding the fabric of the international community. That exceptionalism could be seen in Russia's actions in Ukraine, China's behavior in the South China Sea, the Brazilian government's treatment of its portion of the Amazon basin, and Israel's inexorable disenfranchisement of Palestinians. In all these cases, governments have ignored international norms and practices. They have put themselves above the law.

The greatest sinner in this regard is the United States. The Trump administration did not invent American exceptionalism, but it certainly put the ugliest version of it at the front and center of its foreign policy as it withdrew from international treaties and institutions, violated international law with its military actions and refugee policies, and issued one provocation after another over trade, environment, and human rights.

That exceptionalism has been on florid display during the pandemic as both the president and his core supporters repeatedly assert that they are an exception to the rules that apply to the rest of humanity.

There have been five stages of American exceptionalism in dealing with the coronavirus.

STAGE ONE: It won't happen here.

STAGE TWO: It's happening here, but it's the fault of foreigners.

STAGE THREE: It's happening here, but it won't be as bad as elsewhere so we don't need to take the necessary precautions.

STAGE FOUR: It's happening here, and it might turn out to be a problem, but it's best to address the developing crisis haphazardly rather than at a coordinated federal level.

STAGE FIVE: Uh-oh.

The United States is currently stuck in the uh-oh stage. The presidential election in November 2020 may well remove the immediate problem. But the larger task is the removal of American exceptionalism, the fundamental belief that America is better than other countries and is entitled—by God, by history, by voters—to dictate outcomes around the world rather than work cooperatively on joint solutions.

It will be exceedingly difficult to execute a pandemic pivot if the United States continues to act unilaterally around the world or withdraws behind walls according to a neo-iso-lationist agenda. A pandemic pivot, in short, requires a cooperative United States.

The current US administration is the antithesis of such cooperation. A change in government in Washington would send a strong signal that right-wing authoritarianism is not the wave of the future, that democracy is resilient enough to beat back the attempts by autocratic populists to use the electoral process and a global health crisis to cement their hold on power. The failure of the major right-wing authori-tarian leaders to contain COVID-19—in the United States, Brazil, Russia, and India—has done much to tarnish their reputations and the viability of their ideologies, which are predicated on iron-fisted leadership.

By contrast, as this book suggests, civil society has risen to the challenge of the pandemic. Civic groups all over the world—unions, human rights organizations, peace and justice movements—have pushed back against authoritarian power grabs, organized critical emergency services, and protested against police and military violence. In perhaps the most vivid example, the Black Lives Matter movement inspired millions of people to demonstrate globally against racism and injustice, and issued clear proposals to shift money away from institutions of organized violence and toward human needs. Such a "people's bailout" provides precisely what is needed during this pandemic: health care, unemployment assistance, and better pay and benefits for those with jobs.

On the issue of guns versus butter, the United States needs to make the first move. As the world's biggest spender on the military—more than the next ten countries combined—the United States can single-handedly reverse the dangerous rise in global military expenditures by cutting $350 billion from its defense budget.[245] As the world's leading arms exporter— delivering 76 percent more weapons than runner-up Russia—the United States can lead the world in removing weapons from war and potential conflicts.[246] Re-signing and ratifying the Arms Trade Treaty would be a first step.[247] With enough nuclear weapons to blow up the world many times over, the United States can, with Russia, dramatically reduce the threat of nuclear war, to begin with, by extending the New START arms control treaty.

Shrinking America's overseas military footprint is a key part of reining in American exceptionalism. Closing Cold War–era bases in Europe, mothballing the Africa Command, stopping new base construction on Okinawa: the withdrawal of US troops is an essential part of converting US engagement with the world from primarily military to largely diplomatic. Reducing the flow of arms worldwide and putting funds into peacemaking will also address one of the major root causes of the spike in the number of people seeking safety around the world. Six of the top seven countries of origin for refugees are at war: Syria, Afghanistan, South Sudan, Myanmar, Somalia, and the Democratic Republic of Congo.[248] Demilitarizing borders and closing detention centers as Spain has done would also help address this crisis.

To ensure that the end of US unipolarity doesn't result in an anarchic scramble for power, robust institutions of regional and international security based on multilateral diplomacy, not military, might must fill the gap. The Trump years were marked by a singular hostility toward global institutions. Reversing that trend is essential. America must rejoin the World Health Organization and the UN Human Rights Council, reengage in global climate negotiations, and rejoin and implement the Iran nuclear deal. This is all necessary, but insufficient. Trump, for instance, authorized sanctions against the International Criminal Court (ICC), which had the temerity to propose investigating war crimes in Afghanistan.[249] Immediate removal of these sanctions is critical, but the United States must also re-sign the Rome Treaty and this time actually ratify the accord in the Senate. Membership in the ICC would be a strong signal that the United States is tempering its exceptionalism and finally bringing its conduct into accordance with international law.

Cutting the military budget, closing overseas bases, engaging in serious arms control: all of this will free up considerable resources to meet the great challenge ahead, namely transforming the US economy with a Green New Deal. After all, the climate crisis did not take a coronavirus pause. Unusually high temperatures in the Arctic Ocean have produced a faster-than-expected ice melt in the northern reaches.[250] One-quarter of Bangladesh is underwater, thanks to rising oceans and torrential rains.[251] Extreme heat has helped to create an unprecedented number of large fires in California over the summer.[252]

Dealing with climate change will not come cheap. Becoming carbon-neutral, which the European Union has pledged to do by 2050 and which Norway and Uruguay have more ambitiously promised to do by 2030, will require a massive shift away from dirty energy sources, a huge new infrastructure program that translates this shift into clean transportation and energy-efficient buildings, and a rethinking of the government's role in the economy. A Green New Deal is also the logical response to the economic trends that COVID-19 has accelerated, namely automation and reshoring, for it entails a large-scale Green job-retraining program and a much greater focus on less carbon-intensive manufacturing and local food supply chains.

The Green New Deal is also a vehicle for international engagement. The pandemic has been yet another reminder of how interconnected the world is. Reducing the carbon footprint of only a handful of countries won't save the planet. To make this a collective effort, however, requires richer countries to help speed the transition for poorer countries through debt cancellation and focused assistance so that the latter can leapfrog economically to clean energy technologies.[253] This fair share approach is not charity. It is collective self-interest.

Any truly international effort of this scale requires the United States to find common cause with China. The two countries will disagree about much: trade, human rights, conflicts in East Asia and the Middle East. But there is also much overlap in interests, particularly around climate change and pandemic prevention. If the two major powers can set aside their differences to cooperate for the common good, for instance to push a Global Green New Deal, it would set a powerful example for other countries.

To work at the international level, a Green New Deal requires a rewrite of the rules of the global economy, which has increasingly tilted in favor of corporate interests, particularly around extraction industries like oil, mining, and logging. This rewrite should begin with ending the practice of corporations taking countries to court to overturn their labor, health, and environmental regulations.[254] Then there's the widening global divide between rich and poor—across countries and within countries—that the pandemic has exacerbated. A Global Social Protection Fund that marshals global resources to meet the urgent needs of the world's most vulnerable people can begin to address these gross economic inequities from the bottom up.

The pandemic pivot, in the end, requires a much deeper commitment to democracy, to giving voice to the voiceless. That means strengthening the hand of labor in the workplace, the participation of the undocumented in migration and refugee policy, the involvement of communities most affected by climate change in developing a Green New Deal, and the voices of local peace advocates in building durable ceasefires and peace regimes.[255] It means recognizing that everyone is exceptional in what they can bring to the table and no one is an exception to the rules.

A world of exceptionalisms—America First, China First, India First—is ultimately a world of everyone last, a battle of "all against all" where the effort to seize everything leaves everyone with nothing. The countries that did best against COVID-19 promoted an entirely different mindset of "all for one and one for all." Equity and cooperation are not just nice principles. They're survival strategies.

The pandemic pivot requires a similar choreography: everyone joining hands and moving in concert. Global solidarity in the face of global challenges will not only help achieve the urgent goal of saving the world. It will also help make the world a place worth saving.

PARTICIPANTS

JEFF ABRAMSON is a senior fellow at the Arms Control Association in Washington, DC, and directs the Forum on the Arms Trade, an international network of more than eighty experts working to address the implications of the arms trade, security assistance, and weapons use.

DAVID ADLER is a political economist whose work focuses on the politics of internationalism: how social movements coordinate across borders, and how international institutions aid or impede those efforts. He is the coordinator for the Progressive International movement. Currently based in Florence, Italy, he's a policy leader fellow at the School of Transnational Governance at the European University Institute. He also serves as the policy director for the Democracy in Europe Movement 2025 (DiEM25) and the coordinator of its Green New Deal for Europe campaign. His writing has appeared in the *New York Times*, the *Guardian*, and *Boston Review*.

CHRISTINE AHN is the executive director of Women Cross DMZ, a global movement of women mobilizing for peace in Korea. Based in Hawaii, she's also the co-coordinator of the global feminist campaign Korea Peace Now! Women Mobilizing to End the War.

TOM ATHANASIOU is the executive director of EcoEquity, an activist think tank in California devoted to promoting effective solutions for climate control. He is the author of *Divided Planet: The Ecology of Rich and Poor* and the co-author of *Dead Heat: Global Justice and Global Warming*.

NNIMMO BASSEY is a Nigerian architect, environmental activist, author, and poet, who chaired Friends of the Earth International from 2008 through 2012 and was executive director of Environmental Rights Action for two decades. He was one of *Time* magazine's Heroes of the Environment in 2009. In 2010, Nnimmo was named a laureate of the Right Livelihood Award, and in 2012 he was awarded the Rafto Prize. He serves on the advisory board and is director of the Health of Mother Earth Foundation, an environmental think tank and advocacy organization.

LEO BAUNACH is the director of the International Trade Union Confederation and Global Unions Office in Washington, DC, which advocates for reforming multilateralism and a development model that benefits working people everywhere.

BEN BEACHY is the director of A Living Economy at the Sierra Club in Washington, DC. He has worked on economic policies for over a decade in organizations fighting for workers' rights, climate justice, public health, and self-determination. In 2015 he joined the Sierra Club to help fight corporate trade deals and build power behind people-centered alternatives.

WALDEN BELLO is the co-founder and current senior analyst of the Bangkok-based Focus on the Global South and an international adjunct professor of sociology at the State University of New York at Binghamton. He received the Right Livelihood Award, also known as the Alternative Nobel Prize, in 2003, and was named Outstanding Public Scholar of the International Studies Association in 2008. His newest book is *Counterrevolution: The Global Rise of the Far Right*.

MEDEA BENJAMIN is the co-founder of the women-led peace group CODEPINK and the co-founder of the human rights group Global Exchange. She has been an advocate for social justice for more than forty years. Described as "one of America's most committed—and most effective—fighters for human rights" by *New York Newsday*, and "one of the high-profile leaders of the peace movement" by the *Los Angeles Times*, she was one of one thousand exemplary women from 140 countries nominated to receive the Nobel Peace Prize on behalf of the millions of women who do the essential work of peace worldwide. Her most recent book, *Inside Iran: The Real History and Politics of the Islamic Republic of Iran*, is part of a campaign to prevent a war with Iran and instead promote normal trade and diplomatic relations.

PHYLLIS BENNIS directs the New Internationalism Project at the Institute for Policy Studies, in Washington, DC, focusing on the Middle East, US wars, and UN issues. In 2001, she helped found and remains active with the US Campaign for Palestinian Rights. She works with many anti-war organizations, writing and speaking widely across the United States and around the world as part of the global peace movement. She has served as an informal adviser to several top UN officials on Middle East issues and was twice short-listed to become the UN special rapporteur on human rights in the Occupied Palestinian Territory. She has written and edited eleven books. Among her latest is *Understanding ISIS and the New Global War on Terror: A Primer*, as well as the seventh updated edition of her popular *Understanding the Palestinian-Israeli Conflict*.

SHIKHA BHATTACHARJEE is a lawyer and the research director for Global Labor Justice (GLJ) in Washington, DC. She leads GLJ's work on labor migration in the Persian Gulf and Jordan.

BRID BRENNAN is the coordinator of the Corporate Power project at the Transnational Institute in Amsterdam. She is co-founder of the European Solidarity Centre for the Philippines and, most recently, RESPECT, a Europe-wide anti-racist network for migrant domestic workers.

JORDI CALVO is the vice president of the International Peace Bureau. He is an economist and peace culture, disarmament, and defense economy researcher. He is the coordinator of the Centre Delàs in Barcelona and is an armed conflicts, defense economy, and cooperation lecturer.

JOHN CAVANAGH has been director of the Institute for Policy Studies (IPS) in Washington, DC, since 1999. He directed IPS's Global Economy Program from 1983 to 1997. He is the co-author of twelve books and numerous articles on a wide range of social and economic issues. He sits on the boards of the Congressional Progressive Caucus Center, the International Forum on Globalization, International Labor Rights Forum, the Fund for Constitutional Government, and the New Economy Coalition. He worked as an economist for the United Nations Conference on Trade and Development (1978–81) and the World Health Organization (1981–82). He served on the Civil Society Advisory Committee of the UN Development Program (2000–12).

TOBITA CHOW is the director of Justice Is Global, a special project of People's Action to create a more just and sustainable global economy and defeat right-wing nationalism. Based in Chicago, he is organizing a progressive internationalist alternative to the growing tensions between the United States and China.

WENDELA DE VRIES is a longstanding researcher and campaigner on arms trade and the defense industry for Stop Wapenhandel in Amsterdam and the European Network Against Arms Trade, among others. She recently wrote *Hoe de wapenindustrie probeert te profiteren van de coronacrisis* (How the arms industry tries to profit from the corona crisis) and "Fossil Wars, Arms Trade, and Climate Justice," and is running the petition campaign Geen geld voor nieuwe wapens (No money for new weapons).

FIONA DOVE has been executive director of the Transnational Institute in Amsterdam since 1995. She grew up in South Africa, where she was an anti-apartheid activist from a young age, and later served as a national negotiator and research coordinator for the SA Commercial, Catering and Allied Workers' Union. She serves on the board of De Goede Zaak (Netherlands), the Pluto Educational Trust (UK), the advisory board of the Erasmus Mundus Master in Global Studies coordinated by the University of Leipzig, and the editorial advisory board of the journal *Development in Practice.*

CORAZON VALDEZ FABROS is the vice president of the International Peace Bureau and a core member of the Peace and Security Thematic Circle both at the civil society process at the Asia Europe People's Forum and the ASEAN Civil Society Conference/ASEAN Peoples' Forum. She is lead convener of the STOP the War Coalition (Philippines) and Nuclear Free Pilipinas. She was the former chairperson of the Pacific Concerns Resource Centre (the secretariat of the Nuclear Free and Independent Pacific Movement) and the secretary general of the Nuclear Free Philippines Coalition (NFPC). She is a lawyer by profession, a founding member of the National Union of Peoples' Lawyers, and formerly a business administration professor at the Centro Escolar University in Manila.

CATHY FEINGOLD is the director of the AFL-CIO's International Department in Washington, DC. In 2018, she was elected deputy president of the International Trade Union Confederation, the organization representing two hundred million unionized workers worldwide. She previously directed the AFL-CIO Solidarity Center's work in the Dominican Republic and Haiti, where she worked with local trade union partners to develop innovative campaigns to improve the working conditions of domestic, migrant, and informal economy workers. Her professional experience includes work for the labor movement, large international organizations, small grassroots NGOs, and a foundation. She has written about the impact of economic policies on market women in Nigeria, and, as a Fulbright Scholar in Nicaragua, she researched the impact of structural adjustment policies on women workers.

BRETT FLEISHMAN heads the finance campaign work at 350.org, based in Oakland, California.

JAYATI GHOSH is professor of economics at Jawaharlal Nehru university, New Delhi, and the executive secretary of International Development Economics Associates (IDEAs). She is a regular columnist for several Indian journals and newspapers, a member of the National Knowledge Commission advising the prime minister of India, and is closely involved with a range of progressive organizations and social movements. She is co-recipient of the International Labor Organization's 2010 Decent Work Research prize.

HARRIS GLECKMAN is a senior fellow at the Center for Governance and Sustainability at the University of Massachusetts Boston and director of benchmark environmental consulting. He was a staff member of the UN Centre on Transnational Corporations, head of the New York office of the United Nations Conference on Trade and Development, and an early member of the staff for the 2002 Monterey Conference on Financing for Development.

JACINTA GONZÁLEZ is a senior campaign organizer at Mijente, based in Arizona, and an expert in organizing against immigration enforcement and the criminalization of Latinx and immigrant communities.

SHALMALI GUTTAL is the executive director of Focus on the Global South in Bangkok and has worked with Focus since 1997. She has worked in India, the United States, and mainland Southeast Asia. Her academic background is in the social sciences with particular emphasis on participatory education and qualitative research. Since 1991, she has been researching and writing about economic development, trade and investment, and ecological and social justice issues in Asia—especially the Mekong region and India—with emphasis on people's and women's rights to resources.

THOMAS M. HANNA is research director at The Democracy Collaborative and co-director of the organization's Theory, Policy, and Research Division. His areas of expertise include democratic models of ownership and governance, particularly public and cooperative ownership. His recent publications include *Our Common Wealth: The Return of Public Ownership in the United States* (Manchester University Press, 2018), *The Crisis Next Time: Planning for Public Ownership as an Alternative to Corporate Bank Bailouts* (Next System Project, 2018), and, with Andrew Cumbers, *Constructing the Democratic Public Enterprise* (Democracy Collaborative, 2019). A dual citizen of the United States and the United Kingdom, he has advised the UK Labour Party on democratic public ownership and has served on the advisory board of two European Research Council–funded academic research projects: Transforming Public Policy Through Economic Democracy and Global Remunicipalization and the Post-Neoliberal Turn.

WILLIAM HARTUNG is the director of the Arms and Security Program at the Center for International Policy in Washington, DC, and a senior adviser to the center's Security Assistance Monitor. He is the author of *Prophets of War: Lockheed Martin and the Making of the Military-Industrial Complex* (Nation Books, 2011) and the co-editor, with Miriam Pemberton, of *Lessons from Iraq: Avoiding the Next War* (Paradigm Press, 2008). His previous books include

And Weapons for All (HarperCollins, 1995), a critique of US arms sales policies from the Nixon through the Clinton administrations. From July 2007 through March 2011, he was the director of the Arms and Security Initiative at the New America Foundation. Prior to that, he served as the director of the Arms Trade Resource Center at the World Policy Institute.

RICHARD HEYDARIAN has taught political science at De La Salle University and Ateneo De Manila University, and is an incoming research fellow at National Chengchi University in Taiwan. He is currently resident analyst at GMA Network, a columnist for the Philippine *Daily Inquirer*, and a regular opinion writer for leading global publications. His latest book is *The Rise of Duterte: A Populist Revolt against Elite Democracy* (Palgrave), and he is also the author of *The IndoPacific Age: Trump, China, and the New Global Struggle for Mastery* (Palgrave) as well as *Duterte's Foreign Policy*. He is a regular contributor to the Council on Foreign Relations and Center for Strategic and International Studies in Washington, DC, and has written for and/or been interviewed by Al Jazeera, BBC, Bloomberg, CNN, the *New York Times*, the *Washington Post*, the *Guardian*, the *Wall Street Journal*, *Foreign Affairs*, *Foreign Policy*, and the *Economist*, among other leading global publications.

MEENA JAGANNATH co-founded the Community Justice Project in 2015, and now works as the director of global programs at Movement Law Lab. She is a movement lawyer with an extensive background in activism and international human rights. Prior to coming to Miami, she worked for the Bureau des Avocats Internationaux in Port-au-Prince, Haiti, where she coordinated the Rape Accountability and Prevention Project, which combined direct legal representation with advocacy and capacity building of grassroots women's groups. While using her legal skills to build the power of movements locally in South Florida, she has also brought to bear her international human rights expertise in delegations to the United Nations to elevate US-based human rights issues like police accountability and Stand Your Ground laws to the international level. Meena has published several articles in law journals and other media outlets, and has spoken in numerous academic and conference settings.

BRAMI JEGAN is a Tamil woman and activist in Australia. She works for the Global Strategic Communications Council, a network of climate communicators. She is working on a new project that aims to stigmatize corporate actors profiting from border policing.

REECE JONES teaches in the Department of Geography and Environment at the University of Hawai'i at Mānoa. His latest book is *Violent Borders: Refugees and the Right to Move*.

AKIRA KAWASAKI is an executive committee member of the Tokyo-based NGO Peace Boat and an international steering group member of the 2017 Nobel Peace Prize–winning International Campaign to Abolish Nuclear Weapons (ICAN). He also serves in the Northeast Asia regional secretariat of the Global Partnership for the Prevention of Armed Conflict (GPPAC).

KATE KIZER is the policy director at Win Without War in Washington, DC. She has nearly a decade of experience working on human rights, democratization, and US foreign policy in the Middle East. Kate previously served as the director of policy and advocacy at the Yemen Peace Project and as US advocacy officer for Americans for Democracy and Human Rights in Bahrain.

MICHAEL KLARE is the Five College professor emeritus of peace and world security studies, and director of the Five College Program in Peace and World Security Studies (PAWSS) in Massachusetts. His books include *Resource Wars* (2001), *Blood and Oil* (2004), and *The Race for What's Left* (2012). His articles have appeared in many journals, including *Arms Control Today*, *Bulletin of the Atomic Scientists*, *Current History*, *Foreign Affairs*, *Harper's*, the *Nation*, *Scientific American*, and *Technology Review*. He serves on the board of the Arms Control Association and advises other organizations in the field.

LINDSAY KOSHGARIAN is the program director of the National Priorities Project (NPP), where she oversees NationalPriorities.org. Lindsay's work on the federal budget includes analysis of the federal budget process and politics, military spending, and specifically how federal budget choices for different spending priorities and taxation interact. Prior to joining NPP in 2014, Lindsay was a researcher at the University of Massachusetts Donahue Institute, where she conducted state and regional economic development studies.

LISI KRALL is a professor of economics at the State University of New York, Cortland. She began her academic career as a heterodox labor economist concentrating on gender issues. Her research interests include political economy, human ecology, and the evolution of economic systems. She is currently studying the agricultural revolution and its significance in human social/economic evolution. She has published widely in in diverse journals from the *Cambridge Journal of Economics* to *Behavioral and Brain Sciences*. Her book *Proving Up: Domesticating Land in U.S. History* explores the interconnections of economy, culture, and land.

KAREN HANSEN-KUHN, based in Washington, DC, has been working on trade and economic justice since the beginning of the NAFTA debate.

She has published articles on US trade and agriculture policies, the impacts of US biofuels policies on food security, and women and food crises. She started to learn about the challenges facing farmers as a Peace Corps volunteer in Paraguay, where she worked with a rural cooperative. She was the international coordinator of the Alliance for Responsible Trade (ART), a US multisectoral coalition promoting just and sustainable trade, until 2005. After that, she was policy director at the US office of ActionAid, an international development organization.

EDGARDO LANDER is professor emeritus of sociology at the Central University of Venezuela, a professor at the Universidad Indígena de Venezuela and at the Universidad Andina Simón Bolívar in Quito, a permanent member of the Global Working Group Beyond Development, and one of the organizers of the 2006 World Social Forum in Caracas. In 2017, Edgardo was a founding member of the Plataforma Ciudadana en Defensa de la Constitución (Citizen Platform in Defense of the Constitution) comprised of former Chavistas, who became highly critical of his successor. Edgardo is the author of numerous books and research articles on the environmental limits to industrialization and economic growth, the Left in government in Latin America, post-democratic capitalism, and challenges to Eurocentric epistemologies.

LORA LUMPE is the CEO of the Quincy Institute (QI) for Responsible Statecraft in Washington, DC. Prior to joining QI, she was an advocacy director at the Open Society Foundations (OSF), combatting the corrosive effects of militarism on democracy in the United States and abroad. She is an expert on several aspects of US hyper-militarization, including military budget, arms industry, and weapons sales, military aid and training, child soldiers, gun running, and munitions with disproportionate impact on non-combatants. Prior to OSF, Lora worked for several progressive research and lobby organizations, including the Federation of American Scientists, the Peace Research Institute of Oslo, and the Friends Committee on National Legislation. She has worked on or led a half dozen humanitarian disarmament campaigns—from chemical weapons to cluster munitions. Her books include *Running Guns: The Global Black Market in Small Arms* (2000), *Small Arms Control: Old Weapons, New Issues* (1999), and *The Arms Trade Revealed: A Guide for Investigators and Activists* (1998).

JENS MARTENS has been executive director of Global Policy Forum (New York/Bonn) since its founding in 2004. Since 2011, he has coordinated the international Civil Society Reflection Group on the 2030 Agenda for Sustainable Development. From 2003 to 2009, he was member (2006–9 co-chair) of the Coordinating Committee of Social Watch, a global network of several hundred NGOs working on poverty eradication and social justice. Previously, he was a longstanding member of the executive board of the German NGO World Economy, Ecology and Development (WEED). From 1997 until 2004, he worked at WEED as director of its Programs on International Environment and Development Policy and on Corporate Accountability. Prior to joining the staff at WEED, he worked as a freelance author and adviser for several NGOs and foundations, including the German NGO Forum on Environment and Development, the Friedrich Ebert Foundation, and the Development and Peace Foundation. He has published more than one hundred articles in journals, newspapers, and handbooks, has written several books and studies on development policy and UN reform, and has been co-editor of three books on German UN policy, privatization, and corporate accountability.

TODD MILLER is a journalist based in Tucson, Arizona, and the author, most recently, of *Empire of Borders: The Expansion of the U.S. Border Around the World* (Verso, 2019) as well as the TNI report, More than a Wall.

BRIDGET MOIX serves as Peace Direct's US executive director in Washington, DC. She has worked for twenty years on international peace and conflict issues, with a focus on US foreign policy. Prior to joining Peace Direct's staff, she was part of its founding US board for four years. From 2013 to 2015, Bridget served as atrocity prevention fellow with USAID's Office of Conflict Management and Mitigation. She spent nine years lobbying on US foreign policy and peace issues with the Friends Committee on National Legislation, where she developed and led the Peaceful Prevention of Deadly Conflict program. She has also worked with the Quaker United Nations Office, Oxfam America, American Friends Service Committee, and the World Policy Institute. Bridget directed the Casa de los Amigos in Mexico City, a Quaker center of hospitality and international understanding, from 2006 to 2008. She also worked in Cape Town, South Africa, with the Quaker Peace Centre during her graduate studies internship. Her book *Choosing Peace: Agency and Action in the Midst of War* describes how local and global peacebuilders can work together.

SAMUEL MOYN is Henry R. Luce Professor of Jurisprudence at Yale Law School and professor of history at Yale University. His areas of interest in legal scholarship include international law, human rights, the law of war, and legal thought, in both historical and current perspective. In intellectual history, he has worked on a diverse range of subjects, especially twentieth-century European moral and political theory. He has written several books in his fields of European intellectual history and human rights history, including *The Last Utopia: Human Rights in History* (2010), and edited or co-edited a number of others. His most recent books are

Christian Human Rights (2015, based on Mellon Distinguished Lectures at the University of Pennsylvania in fall 2014) and *Not Enough: Human Rights in an Unequal World* (2018). He is currently working on a new book on the origins and significance of humane war for Farrar, Straus and Giroux. Over the years, he has written in venues such as *Boston Review*, the *Chronicle of Higher Education*, *Dissent*, the *Nation*, the *New Republic*, the *New York Times*, and the *Wall Street Journal*.

AZIZ MUHAMAT is a human rights advocate for migrants, refugees, and asylum seekers, based in Geneva. He is also the 2019 Martin Ennals Award Laureate for Human Rights Defenders and a UN fellow at the Office of the High Commissioner for Human Rights (OHCHR). He has worked as a social worker, journalist, advocate, and vlogger/podcaster, and an author in collaboration with other refugees offshore and inshore on Manus Island. Originally from Darfur in northwestern Sudan, he was held for six years in detention on Manus Island, Papua New Guinea.

JAN-WERNER MÜLLER teaches in the politics department of Princeton University. He has been a member of the School of Historical Studies, Institute of Advanced Study, Princeton, and a visiting fellow at the Collegium Budapest Institute of Advanced Study, Collegium Helsinki, the Institute for Human Sciences in Vienna, the Remarque Institute, New York University, the Center for European Studies, Harvard, as well as the Robert Schuman Centre for Advanced Studies, European University Institute, Florence. He is the author of *Contesting Democracy* (Yale University Press, 2011), *What is Populism?* (University of Pennsylvania Press, 2016), and *Furcht und Freiheit: Für einen anderen Liberalismus* (Suhrkamp, 2019). His public affairs commentary and essays have appeared in the *London Review of Books*, the *New York Review of Books*, *Foreign Affairs*, the *Guardian*, the *New York Times*, and Project Syndicate.

KARIN NANSEN has been the chairperson of Friends of the Earth International since 2016. An environmental justice activist from Uruguay, with a diploma in family farming, Karin is committed to the promotion of food sovereignty and agroecological, diverse, and just food systems. She also campaigns against the expansion of industrial agriculture and corporate control over the food chain, while addressing the root causes of systemic crises, including climate, biodiversity, and food. Karin is a member of the National Coordination of the Native and Local Seeds Network. Working with peasants and rural women has nurtured her understanding of the importance of highlighting the role of women as political subjects in food sovereignty and as leaders in all struggles for environmental and social justice. She was a founding member of Friends of the Earth Uruguay/REDES in 1988.

JOSUE DE LUNA NAVARRO is the New Mexico Fellow at the Institute for Policy Studies. He is the founder of the national UndocuHealth program for United We Dream. In New Mexico, he is the co-founder of the New Mexico Dream Team (NMDT), the largest statewide undocumented-led organization in New Mexico. With the NMDT, he directed a research study in collaboration with the University of New Mexico's TREE Center for Advancing Behavioral Health regarding the health impact of anti-immigrant and racist policies on undocumented youth.

RACHEL ESPLIN ODELL is a PhD candidate in international relations and comparative politics and a member of the MIT Security Studies Program. She is also an international security fellow at Harvard Kennedy School's Belfer Center for Science and International Affairs and a research fellow at the Quincy Institute for Responsible Statecraft in Washington, DC. Her dissertation explains differences in states' interpretation of the international law of the sea and the evolution in those interpretations over time. Her broader research interests include the nature and future of world order, US strategy in the Asia-Pacific region, Chinese foreign policy, and crisis management in Northeast Asia. She previously worked as a research analyst in the Asia Program at the Carnegie Endowment for International Peace.

DIANA OHLBAUM directs the Friends Committee on National Legislation's (FCNL) foreign policy lobbying team in Washington, DC, and leads an effort to replace the current US foreign policy paradigm of military domination and national superiority with a more ethical and effective one based on cooperation and mutual respect. She brings to FCNL nearly two decades of experience on Capitol Hill, where she served as a senior professional staff member of both the House Foreign Affairs Committee and the Senate Foreign Relations Committee, and earlier as an aide to Senator Paul S. Sarbanes (D-MD). During her time as a congressional staff member, Diana coordinated efforts to overhaul the outdated Foreign Assistance Act of 1961, improve oversight of arms sales and security assistance, and promote diplomacy and multilateralism. From 1999 to 2001, she served as deputy director of USAID's Office of Transition Initiatives, a cutting-edge unit designed to advance peace and democracy in priority conflict-prone countries. She also worked as director of public policy for InterAction, an alliance of NGOs engaged in humanitarian relief and international development.

CECILIA OLIVET is a researcher with the Transnational Institute (TNI) in Amsterdam, where she coordinates the Trade and Investment Program. She specializes in the international investment regime. Over the last decade, she has analyzed the impacts of investment treaties and free trade agreements in Latin America, Asia, Africa, and Europe. She is an active member of the Seattle to Brussels (S2B) network. Between 2013 and 2015, Cecilia was a member and chair of the Presidential Commission that audited Ecuador's bilateral investment treaties. She can be reached at ceciliaolivet@tni.org and @CeOlivet.

MÁRTA PARDAVI is co-chair of the Hungarian Helsinki Committee. Márta currently serves on the board of the PILnet Hungary Foundation and the Verzio International Human Rights Documentary Film Festival. Previously she served as board member, and later vice-chair, of the European Council on Refugees and Exiles from 2003 to 2011. She has been awarded the 2018 William D. Zabel Human Rights Award from Human Rights First, the 2019 Civil Rights Defender of the Year Award, and was chosen to be a member of POLITICO 28 Class of 2019.

MIRIAM PEMBERTON is an associate fellow at the Institute for Policy Studies in Washington, DC, and former director of the Peace Economy Transitions Project.

TARSO RAMOS is executive director of Political Research Associates (PRA) in Massachusetts. Under his leadership, PRA has expanded existing lines of research documenting right-wing attacks on reproductive, gender, and racial justice by launching several new initiatives on subjects that include the export of US-style homophobic campaigns abroad, the spread of Islamophobia, and the Right's investment in redefining religious liberty toward discriminatory ends. Before joining PRA, Ramos served as founding director of Western States Center's Racial Justice Program, which works to oppose racist public policy initiatives and support progressive people of color–led organizations. As director of the Wise Use Public Exposure Project in the mid-1990s, he tracked the Right's anti-union and anti-environmental campaigns. As an activist-in-residence at the Barnard Center for Research on Women, Ramos worked on addressing authoritarianism and misogyny as well as examining gender and white supremacy.

ALEX RANDALL is a leading specialist in the connections between climate change, migration, and conflict. He is program manager at the Climate and Migration Coalition in the UK. He has been working on issues around climate, migration, and human rights for fifteen years. He advises a number of key international agencies and governments on their responses to climate-linked migration and displacement. He has also served on the advisory group of the Nansen Initiative and Platform on Disaster Displacement. He has written extensively on climate change and migration for the *Guardian*, *Le Monde diplomatique*, *New Internationalist*, *Prospect*, and numerous other outlets. He is the author of a number of book chapters focusing on the connections between climate change and the rights of refugees and migrants.

ASAD REHMAN is the executive director of War on Want, based in the UK. Prior to that, he was the head of international climate at Friends of the Earth. He has over twenty-five years of experience in the non-government and charity sector. He has served on the boards of Amnesty International UK, Friends of the Earth International, Global Justice Now, and Newham Monitoring Project.

JENNY RICKS, based in South Africa, is the global convener of the Fight Inequality Alliance, a group of human rights, women's rights, environmental, labor, faith-based, and other civil society organizations and movements.

THEA RIOFRANCOS is a 2020 Andrew Carnegie Fellow and assistant professor of political science at Providence College in Rhode Island. She is the author of *Resource Radicals: From Petro-Nationalism to Post-Extractivism in Ecuador* (Duke University Press, 2020) and co-author of *A Planet to Win: Why We Need a Green New Deal* (Verso Books, 2019). She serves on the steering committee of DSA's Ecosocialist Working Group.

MANUEL PEREZ-ROCHA is an associate fellow of the Institute for Policy Studies (IPS) in Washington, DC, and an associate of the Transnational Institute (TNI) in Amsterdam. He is a Mexican national who has led efforts to promote just and sustainable alternative approaches to trade and investment agreements for two decades. Prior to working for IPS's Global Economy Program, he worked with the Mexican Action Network on Free Trade (RMALC) and continues to be a member of that coalition's executive committee. He also worked for the Make Trade Fair campaign of Oxfam International. Some of his latest publications include op-eds in the *Nation* and the *New York Times*.

ERIKA GUEVARA ROSAS is a Mexican-American human rights lawyer and feminist activist who currently serves as the Americas director at Amnesty International, where she leads the organization's human rights work across the continent. She brings more than twenty years of experience in social and gender justice, human rights, and philanthropy.

WOLFRAM SCHAFFAR is a professor of Japanese studies at the University of Tübingen and an associated researcher in the Department of Southeast Asian Studies, University of Passau. From 2010 until 2018, he was a professor of development studies and political science in the Department of Development Studies at the University of Vienna. Prior to this, he was affiliated with the University of Bonn, Chulalongkorn University in Bangkok, and the Royal Netherlands Institute of Southeast Asian and Caribbean Studies (KITLV) in Leiden, Netherlands. His fields of interest are state theory of the Global South, social movements, new constitutionalism, and democratization processes, as well as the new authoritarianism.

BASAV SEN is the Climate Justice Project director at the Institute for Policy Studies (IPS) in Washington, DC, where he focuses on climate solutions at the national, state, and local levels that address racial, economic, gender, and other forms of inequality. Prior to joining IPS, Basav worked for about eleven years as a strategic corporate campaign researcher at the United Food and Commercial Workers (UFCW). He has also had experience as a campaigner on the World Bank, International Monetary Fund (IMF), and global finance and trade issues.

COUMBA TOURÉ, a writer and storyteller, was born and raised between Mali and Senegal. She is the co-coordinator of Africans Rising for Justice, Peace and Dignity and a board member of TrustAfrica. She publishes children's stories and organizes art events targeting children's minds through Falia. She also designs popular education programs with a focus to impact women and children. She has extensive experience in facilitating meetings internationally, engaging young people, designing, implementing, and evaluating training programs to promote human rights, especially those of women. Coumba has promoted social entrepreneurship through her work with Ashoka for the past ten years. She has worked with organizations such as the Institute for Popular Education in Mali, the 21st Century Youth Leadership Movement in Selma, Alabama, and the Youth for Environmental Sanity in Santa Cruz, California. She is a member of the African Feminist Forum and the Per Ankh collective.

SANHO TREE is a fellow at the Institute for Policy Studies in Washington, DC, and has been director of its Drug Policy Project since 1998. A former military and diplomatic historian, his current work encompasses the reform of both international and domestic drug policies by promoting alternatives to the failed prohibitionist model. He previously collaborated with Gar Alperovitz on *The Decision to Use the Atomic Bomb and the Architecture of an American Myth* (Knopf, 1995). He was also associate editor of *CovertAction Quarterly*, an award-winning magazine of investigative journalism, and he worked at the International Human Rights Law Group in the late 1980s. Currently, he serves on the board of the Andean Information Network.

JORDI VAQUER is the director for Global Foresight and Analysis at the Open Society Foundations. Previously, he was the Open Society Foundations regional director for Europe and a co-director of the Open Society

Initiative for Europe. He is an affiliated lecturer at the Barcelona Institute for International Affairs and a regular contributor to Spanish media on international affairs and EU politics. Before joining the Open Society Foundations, he was director of the Barcelona Centre for International Affairs, one of southern Europe's most influential international relations think tanks.

DAVID VINE is professor of anthropology at American University in Washington, DC, and a board member of the Costs of War Project. David is the author of several books about war and peace including a new book, *The United States of War: A Global History of America's Endless Conflicts, from Columbus to the Islamic State.*

JAKE WERNER, one of the co-founders of Justice Is Global, is a historian of modern China. He is director of policy and political research at PrestonWerner Ventures and is an incoming research fellow at the Global Development Policy Center at Boston University. His work has appeared in the *Nation, Foreign Policy,* and *Made in China.*

CINDY WIESNER is the executive director of Grassroots Global Justice Alliance in Florida. A twenty-five-year veteran of the social justice movement in the United States and internationally, she helped co-found the Climate Justice Alliance and has played a leadership role in the Peoples Climate Movement that organized the massive mobilizations in New York, Washington, DC, and San Francisco in recent years, and is an adviser to Groundswell's Liberation Fund. She started organizing with HERE Local 2850 in Oakland, California, and went on to become the director of organizing for People Organizing to Win Employment Rights in San Francisco and an organizer and board member for generationFIVE. She has also been a consultant for Men Overcoming Violence Everywhere and Mujeres Unidas y Activas. She previously worked as leadership development director of the Miami Workers Center and represented the group as a member of the US Social Forum National Planning Committee. She has been active in many movement building initiatives over the years, including World March of Women, Social Movement Assemblies, International Council of the World Social Forum, Fight Against the FTAA, UNITY, Building Equity and Alignment Initiative, and, currently, It Takes Roots and the Rising Majority.

NOTES

1   Ole Benedictow, "The Black Death: The Greatest Catastrophe Ever," *History Today*, March 3, 2005; https://www.historytoday.com/archive/black-death-greatest-catastrophe-ever.

2   "Spanish Flu," History.com, May 19, 2020; https://www.history.com/topics/world-war-i/1918-flu-pandemic.

3   Edward Wong, Julian E. Barnes, and Zolan Kanno-Youngs, "Local Officials in China Hid Coronavirus Dangers From Beijing, U.S. Agencies Find," *The New York Times*, August 19, 2020; https://www.nytimes.com/2020/08/19/world/asia/china-coronavirus-beijing-trump.html.

4   Natalie Colarossi, "In February, the CDC Outlined a Chilling 'Hypothetical' Scenario about How the Coronavirus Could Spread in the US. It Was Shockingly Close to Reality," *Business Insider*, April 18, 2020; https://www.businessinsider.com/cdc-outline-for-coronavirus-spread-in-february-pars-with-reality-2020-4.

5   Alexandra Brzozowski, "UN Chief Calls for 'Immediate Global Ceasefire' amid COVID-19 Pandemic," EurActiv, March 24, 2020; https://www.euractiv.com/section/global-europe/news/un-chief-calls-for-immediate-global-ceasefire-amid-covid-19-pandemic/.

6   "The People's Vaccine," UNAIDS, May 14, 2020; https://www.unaids.org/en/resources/presscentre/pressreleaseandstatementarchive/2020/may/20200514_covid19-vaccine.

7   Chris Mooney, Brady Dennis, and John Muyskens, "Global Emissions Plunged an Unprecedented 17 Percent during the Coronavirus Pandemic," *The Washington Post*, May 19, 2020; https://www.washingtonpost.com/climate-environment/2020/05/19/greenhouse-emissions-coronavirus/?arc404=true.

8   Morgan Chalfant and Brett Samuels, "Trump Leans into Executive Action, Looking for 2020 Boost," *The Hill*, August 6, 2020; https://thehill.com/homenews/administration/510803-trump-leans-into-executive-action-looking-for-2020-boost; Emma Newburger, "Trump Lifts Obama-Era Regulations on Methane, a Potent Climate-Warming Gas," CNBC, August 13, 2020; https://www.cnbc.com/2020/08/13/trump-lifts-obama-era-regulations-on-climate-changing-methane-gas.html; Brian

Bennett, "President Trump Has Blocked New Legal Immigrants. Here's Where Else He's Clamped Down on Immigration During the Coronavirus Outbreak," *Time*, April 22, 2020; https://time.com/5825141/president-trump-immigration-coronavirus/.

9   "Air Pollution," World Health Organization; https://www.who.int/health-topics/air-pollution#tab=tab_1; Kelly McLaughlin, "India's Air Quality Has Improved So Much Since the Country Went on Coronavirus Lockdown Citizens Can Now See the Himalayas for the First Time in 30 Years," April 13, 2020; https://www.insider.com/himalayas-seen-from-india-pollution-drop-coronavirus-lockdown-2020-4; Drew Kann, "Coronavirus: LA's Air, Usually Terrible, Is Best in the World," *The Mercury News*, April 7, 2020; https://www.mercurynews.com/2020/04/07/coronavirus-las-air-usually-terrible-is-best-in-the-world/.

10   Terrence McCoy, "As Humans Stay Indoors, Wild Animals Take Back What Was Once Theirs," *The Washington Post*, April 15, 2020; https://www.washingtonpost.com/world/the_americas/coronavirus-wild-animals-wales-goats-barcelona-boars-brazil-turtles/2020/04/14/30057b2c-7a71-11ea-b6ff-597f170df8f8_story.html.

11   The World Bank, "Pandemic, Recession: The Global Economy in Crisis," June 8 2020; https://www.worldbank.org/en/publication/global-economic-prospects.

12   Damian Carrington and Niko Kommenda, "Air Pollution in China Back to Pre-Covid Levels and Europe May Follow," *The Guardian*, June 3, 2020; https://www.theguardian.com/environment/2020/jun/03/air-pollution-in-china-back-to-pre-covid-levels-and-europe-may-follow.

13   Andrew Freedman and Chris Mooney, "Earth's Carbon Dioxide Levels Hit Record High, Despite Coronavirus-Related Emissions Drop," *The Washington Post*, June 4, 2020; https://www.washingtonpost.com/weather/2020/06/04/carbon-dioxide-record-2020/.

14   Karin Kirk, "Coronavirus Pandemic Leads to Profound Cutbacks in Fossil Fuel Use," *Yale Climate Connections*, April 30, 2020; https://yaleclimateconnections.org/2020/04/coronavirus-pandemic-leads-to-profound-cutbacks-in-fossil-fuel-use/.

15   Rystad Energy, "2020's Oil Demand Recovery Seen a Bit Slower, 2021 Demand Downgraded," May 29, 2020; https://www.rystadenergy.com/newsevents/news/press-releases/covid-19-weekly-update-2020s-oil-demand-recovery-seen-a-bit-slower-2021-demand-downgraded/.

16   Macrotrends, "Crude Oil Prices-70 Year Historical Chart," https://www.macrotrends.net/1369/crude-oil-price-history-chart; Camila Domonoske, "U.S. Oil Prices Fall Below Zero For The First Time In History," NPR, April 21, 2020; https://www.npr.org/2020/04/21/839522390/u-s-oil-prices-fall-below-zero-for-the-first-time-in-history.

17   Clifford Krauss, "Oil Nations, Prodded by Trump, Reach Deal to Slash Production," *The New York Times*, April 12, 2020; https://www.nytimes.com/2020/04/12/business/energy-environment/opec-russia-saudi-arabia-oil-coronavirus.html.

18   Carbon Tracker, "2020 Vision: Why You Should See the Fossil Fuel Peak Coming," September 10, 2018; https://carbontracker.org/reports/2020-vision-why-you-should-see-the-fossil-fuel-peak-coming/.

19   Benjamin Storrow, "Global CO2 Has Risen for a Century. That Appears To Be Over," *E & E News*, June 1, 2020; https://www.eenews.net/stories/1063286379.

20   Matt McGrath, "Coronavirus: Air pollution and CO2 Fall Rapidly as Virus

Spreads," BBC, March 19, 2020; https://www.bbc.com/news/science-environ-ment-51944780.

21   Rebecca Elliott and Christopher Matthews, "Oil and Gas Bankruptcies Grow as Investors Lose Appetite for Shale," *The Wall Street Journal*, August 30, 2019; https://www.wsj.com/articles/oil-and-gas-bankruptcies-grow-as-investors-lose-appetite-for-shale-11567157401; Daniel Moritz-Rabson, "Eleven Coal Companies Have Filed for Bankruptcy Since Trump Took Office," *Newsweek*, October 30, 2019; https://www.newsweek.com/eight-coal-companies-have-filed-bankruptcy-since-trump-took-office-1468734.

22   Trefis Team, "$70 Billion: How much Exxon Mobil Will Shrink in 2020," *Forbes*, May 15, 2020; https://www.forbes.com/sites/greatspeculations/2020/05/15/70-billion-how-much-exxon-mobil-will-shrink-in-2020/#2c242adf73be; Dion Rabouin, "Why the Dow Jones Shook Up Its Members," *Axios*, August 25, 2020; https://www.axios.com/dow-jones-changes-members-pfizer-exxon-raytheon-6ab831cd-a9bf-47f2-9788-10f8c59d1998.html.

23   Rebecca Beitsch and Rachel Frazin, "Oil Companies Get $1.9B in Tax Benefits under Stimulus," *The Hill*, May 15, 2020; https://thehill.com/policy/energy-environment/498065-overnight-energy-analysis-oil-companies-have-received-19b-in-tax.

24   Christina Larson, "How the Internet Is Powering the Fight against Beijing's Dirty Air," *The Guardian*, April 10, 2012; https://www.theguardian.com/environment/2012/apr/10/internet-beijing-dirty-air-pollution.

25   Climate & Clean Air Coalition, "Beijing's Air Quality Improvements Are a Model for Other Cities," March 9, 2019; https://www.ccacoalition.org/en/news/beijing%E2%80%99s-air-quality-improvements-are-model-other-cities.

26   Feargus O'Sullivan, "Europe's Cities Are Making Less Room for Cars After Coronavirus," *Bloomberg CityLab*, April 22, 2020; https://www.bloomberg.com/news/articles/2020-04-22/a-car-free-blueprint-for-city-life-after-lockdown.

27   Jack Ewing, "The Pandemic Will Permanently Change the Auto Industry," *The New York Times*, May 13, 2020; https://www.nytimes.com/2020/05/13/business/auto-industry-pandemic.html.

28   Sabrina Kessler, "Coronavirus Pandemic Fuels Comeback of Cars," *Deutsche Welle*, June 10, 2020; https://www.dw.com/en/coronavirus-pandemic-fuels-comeback-of-cars/a-53759607.

29   World Bank, "Most Commodity Prices to Drop in 2020 As Coronavirus Depresses Demand and Disrupts Supply," April 23, 2020; https://www.worldbank.org/en/news/press-release/2020/04/23/most-commodity-prices-to-drop-in-2020-as-coronavirus-depresses-demand-and-disrupts-supply.

30   Congressional Research Service, "Export Restrictions in Response to the COVID-19 Pandemic," August 25, 2020; https://crsreports.congress.gov/product/pdf/IF/IF11551.

31   Beth Gardiner, "How Renewable Energy Could Emerge on Top After the Pandemic," *YaleEnvironment360*, May 12, 2020; https://e360.yale.edu/features/how-renewable-energy-could-emerge-on-top-after-the-pandemic.

32   Heymi Bahar, "The Coronavirus Pandemic Could Derail Renewable Energy's Progress. Governments Can Help," International Energy Agency, April 4, 2020; https://www.iea.org/commentaries/the-coronavirus-pandemic-could-derail-renewable-energy-s-progress-governments-can-help.

33 Nichola Groom, "Despite Pandemic, New U.S. Solar Capacity Will Grow 33% in 2020," Reuters, June 11, 2020; https://www.reuters.com/article/us-usa-solar-report/despite-pandemic-new-u-s-solar-capacity-will-grow-33-in-2020-idUSKBN23I-oHL.

34 Lisa Cox, "Australia Could Get 90% of Electricity from Renewables by 2040 with No Price Increase," *The Guardian*, April 28, 2020; https://www.theguardian.com/australia-news/2020/apr/29/australia-could-get-90-of-electricity-from-renewables-by-2040-with-no-price-increase; "Renewables Make Up Over Half of Germany's Power Mix," *Deutsche Welle*, April 1, 2020; https://www.dw.com/en/renewables-make-up-over-half-of-germanys-power-mix/a-52986924?maca=en-VAM_volltext_ecowatch-28485-html-copypaste.

35 Jason Wilson, "Eco-Fascism Is Undergoing a Revival in the Fetid Culture of the Extreme Right," *The Guardian*, March 19, 2019; https://www.theguardian.com/world/commentisfree/2019/mar/20/eco-fascism-is-undergoing-a-revival-in-the-fetid-culture-of-the-extreme-right.

36 Sarah Murawski, "Time to Resolve Debt Issues in the Global South," Transnational Institute, April 17, 2020; https://www.tni.org/en/article/time-to-resolve-debt-issues-in-the-global-south.

37 Chuck Collins, Omar Ocampo, and Sophia Paslaski, *Billionaire Bonanza 2020*, Institute for Policy Studies, April 23, 2020; https://ips-dc.org/billionaire-bonanza-2020/.

38 Elizabeth Kolbert, "How Iceland Beat the Coronavirus," *The New Yorker*, June 1, 2020; https://www.newyorker.com/magazine/2020/06/08/how-iceland-beat-the-coronavirus; John Feffer, "In New Zealand, David Confronts 2 Goliaths," *The Nation*, May 25, 2020; https://www.thenation.com/article/world/new-zealand-extremism-coronavirus/.

39 For instance, 350.org's "People, Not Polluters" campaign, https://350.org/people-not-polluters/.

40 Uri Friedman, "The Coronavirus-Denial Movement Now Has a Leader," *The Atlantic*, March 27, 2020; https://www.theatlantic.com/politics/archive/2020/03/bolsonaro-coronavirus-denial-brazil-trump/608926/.

41 People's Bailout, https://thepeoplesbailout.org/.

42 David Roberts, "There's Now an Official Green New Deal. Here's What's in It," *Vox*, February 7, 2019; https://www.vox.com/energy-and-environment/2019/2/7/18211709/green-new-deal-resolution-alexandria-ocasio-cortez-markey.

43 Simon Brandon, "Europe Must Overcome These 3 Challenges to Seal the European Green Deal," World Economic Forum, June 11, 2020; https://www.weforum.org/agenda/2020/06/3-challenges-covid-19-european-green-deal-european-commission/.

44 John Feffer, "A Progressive Victory over the Coronavirus," Foreign Policy In Focus, April 22, 2020; https://fpif.org/a-progressive-victory-over-the-coronavirus/.

45 Ben Beachy, *Millions of Good Jobs: A Plan for Economic Renewal*, Sierra Club, May 2020; https://www.sierraclub.org/sites/www.sierraclub.org/files/economic-renewal.pdf.

46 Robert Samuelson, "How 'Long Economic Waves' Could Save Capitalism," *The Washington Post*, June 14, 2020; https://www.washingtonpost.com/opinions/how-long-economic-waves-could-save-the-recovery/2020/06/14/586478c0-acdf-11ea-9063-e69bd6520940_story.html.

47 Harald Fuhr, "The Global South's Contribution to the Climate Crisis—and Its Potential Solutions," OECD Development Matters, June 20, 2019; https://oecd-development-matters.org/2019/06/20/the-global-souths-contribution-to-the-climate-crisis-and-its-potential-solutions/.

48 Climate Equity Reference Calculator; https://calculator.climateequityreference.org/.

49 War on Want, "The UK's Climate Fair Share Infographic," March 2020; https://waronwant.org/resources/uks-climate-fair-share-infographic.

50 Global Green New Deal; https://www.globalgnd.org.

51 Adnan Seric, Holger Görg, Saskia Mösle, and Michael Windisch, "Managing COVID-19: How the Pandemic Disrupts Global Value Chains," World Economic Forum, April 27, 2020; https://www.weforum.org/agenda/2020/04/covid-19-pandemic-disrupts-global-value-chains/; Jason Alexander and Lawrence Keyler, "Coronavirus Pandemic Hinders Global Automotive Supply Chains," RSM, March 31, 2020; https://rsmus.com/what-we-do/industries/industrials/automotive/coronavirus-pandemic-hinders-global-automotive-supply-chains.html; Caroline Baum, "Could Apple Be the Canary in the Coal Mine for Coronavirus?" MarketWatch, February 19, 2020; https://www.marketwatch.com/story/could-apple-be-the-canary-in-the-coal-mine-for-coronavirus-2020-02-19; Simone McCarthy, "Coronavirus Could Cause Global Medicine Shortages as China's Factory Closures Hit Supply Chains," South China Morning Post, March 4, 2020; https://www.scmp.com/news/china/society/article/3064989/coronavirus-could-cause-global-medicine-shortages-chinas-factory.

52 Ned Temko, "No Jobs, so What Future? Half the World's Workforce on the Edge," Christian Science Monitor, May 6, 2020; https://www.csmonitor.com/World/2020/0506/No-jobs-so-what-future-Half-the-world-s-workforce-on-the-edge.

53 World Bank, "The Global Economic Outlook During the COVID-19 Pandemic: A Changed World," June 8, 2020; https://www.worldbank.org/en/news/feature/2020/06/08/the-global-economic-outlook-during-the-covid-19-pandemic-a-changed-world.

54 Gita Gopinath, "The Great Lockdown: Worst Economic Downturn Since the Great Depression," IMFBlog, April 14, 2020; https://blogs.imf.org/2020/04/14/the-great-lockdown-worst-economic-downturn-since-the-great-depression/.

55 Andrew Van Dam, "The U.S. Has Thrown More than $6 Trillion at the Coronavirus Crisis. That Number Could Grow," The Washington Post, April 15, 2020; https://www.washingtonpost.com/business/2020/04/15/coronavirus-economy-6-trillion/; Swaha Pattanaik, "Does $20 Trillion Buy Much Inflation?" Reuters, August 11, 2020; https://www.reuters.com/article/us-global-economy-inflation-breakingview/breakingviews-does-20-trillion-buy-much-inflation-idUSKCN25711P.

56 Michael Birnbaum and Karla Adam, "Europe Seeks to Limit Coronavirus Crisis with Unprecedented Offers to Pay Private-Sector Salaries," The Washington Post, March 24, 2020; https://www.washingtonpost.com/world/europe/europe-seeks-to-limit-coronavirus-crisis-with-unprecedented-offers-to-pay-private-sector-salaries/2020/03/24/1f099a5a-6abe-11ea-b199-3a9799c54512_story.html.

57 "The Steam Has Gone out of Globalization," The Economist, January 24, 2019; https://www.economist.com/leaders/2019/01/24/the-steam-has-gone-out-of-globalisation.

58　"Globalization: Myth and Reality," *Harvard Business Review*, February 24, 2017; OECD, "Global Value Chains and Trade," https://www.oecd.org/trade/topics/global-value-chains-and-trade/.

59　Keith Bradsher, "China Dominates Medical Supplies, in this Outbreak and the Next," *The New York Times*, July 5, 2020; https://www.nytimes.com/2020/07/05/business/china-medical-supplies.html.

60　K. De Backer et al., "Industrial Robotics and the Global Organisation of Production," OECD Science, Technology and Industry Working Papers, No. 2018/03; https://doi.org/10.1787/dd98ff58-en.

61　Melissa Repko and Amelia Lucas, "The Meat Supply Chain Is Broken. Here's Why Shortages Are Likely to Last during the Coronavirus Pandemic," CNBC, May 20, 2020; https://www.cnbc.com/2020/05/07/heres-why-meat-shortages-are-likely-to-last-during-the-pandemic.html.

62　Andrea Shalal, "80 Countries Are Hoarding Medical Supplies—Here's Why It Damages the Global Response to COVID-19," World Economic Forum, April 24, 2020; https://www.weforum.org/agenda/2020/04/wto-report-80-countries-limiting-exports-medical-supplies/.

63　Valentina Romel, "Pandemic Causes 'Unprecedented' Fall in Global Trade," *Financial Times*, June 25, 2020; https://www.ft.com/content/d870d304-9ee8-4699-ae02-cf-4e1c488d2a.

64　World Trade Organization, "Trade Falls Steeply in First Half of 2020," June 22, 2020; https://www.wto.org/english/news_e/pres20_e/pr858_e.htmn.

65　Sidley, "The Basics of Bilateral Investment Treaties," https://www.sidley.com/en/global/services/global-arbitration-trade-and-advocacy/investment-treaty-arbitration/sub-pages/the-basics-of-bilateral-investment-treaties/.

66　Sarah Babbage, "What Trump, Johnson Want From U.S.-U.K. Trade Deal," *The Washington Post*, June 11, 2020; https://www.washingtonpost.com/business/what-trump-johnson-want-from-us-uk-trade-deal/2020/06/10/e116d732-ab75-11ea-a43b-be9f6494a87d_story.html.

67　Karen Hansen-Kuhn and Catherine Gatundu, "U.S.-Kenya FTA and the Rights to Land and Food," Institute for Agriculture and Trade Policy, May 5, 2020; https://www.iatp.org/blog/202005/us-kenya-fta-and-rights-land-and-food; Stephanie Senet, "EU-Mercosur Deal Will Have Devastating Impact on Climate, NGOs Warn," EurActiv, July 2, 2020; https://www.euractiv.com/section/economy-jobs/news/eu-mercosur-deal-will-have-devastating-impact-on-climate-ngos-warn/.

68　"Coronavirus: Travel Restrictions, Border Shutdowns by Country," Al Jazeera, June 3, 2020; https://www.aljazeera.com/news/2020/03/coronavirus-travel-restrictions-border-shutdowns-country-200318091505922.html.

69　"John Magufuli Declares Tanzania Free of Covid-19," BBC, June 8, 2020; https://www.bbc.com/news/world-africa-52966016.

70　Christopher Miller, "This Leader Has Banned His Doctors From Saying The Word 'Coronavirus'—And Refuses To Admit There Are Any Cases," Buzzfeed, May 1, 2020; https://www.buzzfeednews.com/article/christopherm51/coronavirus-turkmenistan.

71　UNDP, "Coronavirus vs. inequality," https://feature.undp.org/coronavirus-vs-inequality/.

72　ILO, "As Jobs Crisis Deepens, ILO Warns of Uncertain and Incomplete Labour

Market Recovery," June 30, 2020; https://www.ilo.org/global/about-the-ilo/news-room/news/WCMS_749398/lang--en/index.htm.

73   Brett Molina, "Jeff Bezos Could Become World's First Trillionaire, and Many People Aren't Happy about It," *USAToday*, May 14, 2020; https://www.usatoday.com/story/tech/2020/05/14/jeff-bezos-worlds-first-trillionaire-sparks-heated-debate/5189161002/.

74   Ashley Viens, "Ranked: The Richest Countries in the World," *Visual Capitalist*, May 24, 2019; https://www.visualcapitalist.com/richest-countries-in-world/.

75   Charles Lane, "The New Deal as Raw Deal for Blacks in Segregated Communities," *The Washington Post*, May 25, 2017; https://www.washingtonpost.com/opinions/the-new-deal-as-raw-deal-for-blacks-in-segregated-communities/2017/05/25/07416b-ba-080a-11e7-a15f-a58d4a988474_story.html; Juan Perea, "The Echoes of Slavery: Recognizing the Racist Origins of the Agricultural and Domestic Worker Exclusion from the National Labor Relations Act," 72 OHIO ST. L.J.1 95 (2011); https://lawecommons.luc.edu/cgi/viewcontent.cgi?article=1150&context=facpubs.

76   "David Harvey at The Future is Public Conference in Amsterdam," YouTube, December 23, 2019; https://www.youtube.com/watch?v=ngxc_tJkcfY.

77   "Rodrigo Duterte's Lawless War on Drugs Is Wildly Popular," *The Economist*, February 20, 2020; https://www.economist.com/briefing/2020/02/20/rodrigo-duter-tes-lawless-war-on-drugs-is-wildly-popular.

78   International Center for Not-for-Profit Law, "COVID-19 Civic Freedom Tracker," https://www.icnl.org/covid19tracker/?location=&issue=5&date=&type.

79   "Global Democracy Has Another Bad Year," *The Economist*, January 22, 2020; https://www.economist.com/graphic-detail/2020/01/22/global-democracy-has-an-other-bad-year.

80   Sarah Repucci, "A Leaderless Struggle for Democracy," Freedom House, March 4, 2020; https://freedomhouse.org/report/freedom-world/2020/leaderless-struggle-de-mocracy.

81   World Justice Project, "Rule of Law Index 2020," https://worldjusticeproject.org/sites/default/files/documents/WJP-ROLI-2020-Online_0.pdf.

82   Fred DeVeaux, "Democracy Perception Index–2020," Dalia, June 15, 2020; https://daliaresearch.com/blog/democracy-perception-index-2020/.

83   Anna Lührmann and Staffan I. Lindberg, "A Third Wave of Autocratization Is Here: What Is New about It?" *Democratization*, Vol 26, no. 7 (2019); https://www.tandfonline.com/doi/full/10.1080/13510347.2019.1582029.

84   "List of George Floyd Protests outside the United States," Wikipedia; https://en.wikipedia.org/wiki/List_of_George_Floyd_protests_outside_the_United_States.

85   Naomi O'Leary, "Calls for EU to Act as NGO Deems Hungary No Longer a Democracy," *The Irish Times*, May 7, 2020; https://www.irishtimes.com/news/world/europe/calls-for-eu-to-act-as-ngo-deems-hungary-no-longer-a-democracy-1.4247748.

86   Ishaan Tharoor, "A Journalist's Conviction Spells Trouble for Democracy in the Philippines," *The Washington Post*, June 23, 2020; https://www.washingtonpost.com/world/2020/06/23/maria-ressa-philippines-democracy-duterte/.

87   "Mood of the Nation: PM Modi Still King of Indian politics with 78 Percent Approval Rating," *India Today*, August 7, 2020; https://www.indiatoday.in/magazine/india/story/20200817-mood-of-the-nation-pm-modi-still-king-of-indian-politics-with-78-per-cent-approval-rating-1708943-2020-08-07; Jean Dreze, "India Is in

Denial about the COVID-19 Crisis," *Scientific American*, August 25, 2020; https://www.scientificamerican.com/article/india-is-in-denial-about-the-covid-19-crisis/; Kathryn Salam, "Kashmir, One Year Later," *Foreign Policy*, August 4, 2020; https://foreignpolicy.com/2020/08/04/kashmir-article-370-blackout-arrest-covid-pandemic-modi/; Siobhán O'Grady, "Trump Stays Quiet on Modi Crackdown," *The Washington Post*, December 19, 2019; https://www.washingtonpost.com/world/2019/12/19/trump-stays-quiet-modis-crackdown/.

88   Leah Sottile, "The Chaos Agents," *The New York Times*, August 19, 2020; https://www.nytimes.com/interactive/2020/08/19/magazine/boogaloo.html.

89   Jeremy Howard, "Simple DIY Masks Could Help Flatten the Curve. We Should All Wear Them in Public," *The Washington Post*, March 28, 2020; https://www.washingtonpost.com/outlook/2020/03/28/masks-all-coronavirus/.

90   #Masks4All; https://masks4all.org/.

91   International Institute for Democracy and Electoral Assistance, "Global Overview of COVID-19: Impact on Elections," accessed August 29, 2020; https://www.idea.int/news-media/multimedia-reports/global-overview-covid-19-impact-elections.

92   Justin McCurry, "South Korea's Ruling Party Wins Election Landslide amid Coronavirus Outbreak," *The Guardian*, April 15, 2020; https://www.theguardian.com/world/2020/apr/16/south-koreas-ruling-party-wins-election-landslide-amid-coronavirus-outbreak.

93   Matthew Luxmoore, "Election Monitors Find 'Unprecedented' Levels Of Fraud In Russian Vote On Extending Putin's Rule," RFE/RL, July 3, 2020; https://www.rferl.org/a/election-monitors-find-unprecedented-levels-of-fraud-in-russian-vote-on-extending-putin-s-rule/30704791.html.

94   Iolanda Fonseca, "Brazil Will Establish Post-Pandemic Minimum Income Program, Says Economy Minister," *The Rio Times*, June 10, 2020; https://riotimesonline.com/brazil-news/brazil/brazils-government-to-establish-post-pandemic-minimum-income-program-says-economy-minister-2/.

95   Emma O'Dwyer, "COVID-19 mutual aid groups have the potential to increase intergroup solidarity—but can they actually do so?" London School of Economics, June 23, 2020; https://blogs.lse.ac.uk/politicsandpolicy/covid19-mutual-aid-solidarity/.

96   Maziyar Ghiabi, "Mutual Aid and Solidarity in Iran during the COVID-19 Pandemic," Middle East Report Online, April 17, 2020; https://merip.org/2020/04/mutual-aid-and-solidarity-in-iran-during-the-covid-19-pandemic/.

97   "Refugees at Highest Ever Level, Reaching 65m, Says UN," BBC, June 20, 2016; https://www.bbc.com/news/world-36573082.

98   UNHCR, "Figures at a Glance," June 18, 2020, https://www.unhcr.org/ph/figures-at-a-glance.

99   "COVID-19: Agencies Temporarily Suspend Refugee Resettlement Travel," *UN News*, March 17, 2020; https://news.un.org/en/story/2020/03/1059602.

100 David Kamiab Hesari, Marrium Habib, Muhammad Zaman, and Clarissa Prazeres da Costa, "Germany and COVID-19: What About the Refugees?" *Global Health Now*, June 2, 2020; https://www.globalhealthnow.org/2020-06/germany-and-covid-19-what-about-refugees.

101 Daniel Cassady, "Coronavirus Runs Rampant In Virginia ICE Detention Facility," *Forbes*, July 23, 2020; https://www.forbes.com/sites/danielcassady/2020/07/23/coro-

navirus-runs-rampant-in-virginia-ice-detention-facility/#6002ef523b37.

102   Chantal da Silva, "Portugal Is Giving Citizenship Rights to Migrants and Asylum Seekers so They Can Access Health Care Amid Coronavirus Outbreak," *Newsweek*, May 11, 2020; https://www.newsweek.com/portugal-citizenship-rights-migrants-asylum-seekers-health-care-coronavirus-1503178.

103   Wudan Yan, "Only One Country Offers Universal Health Care To All Migrants," NPR, March 31, 2016; https://www.npr.org/sections/goatsandsoda/2016/03/31/469608931/only-one-country-offers-universal-health-care-to-undocumented-migrants.

104   Patricia Mazzei, "Florida's Coronavirus Spike is Ravaging Migrant Farmworkers," *The New York Times*, June 18, 2020; https://www.nytimes.com/2020/06/18/us/florida-coronavirus-immokalee-farmworkers.html; Rebecca Staudenmaier, "Germany's Meat industry under Fire after COVID-19 Outbreaks," *Deutsche Welle*, May 19, 2020; https://www.dw.com/en/germanys-meat-industry-under-fire-after-covid-19-outbreaks/a-53502751; Jesse Yeung and Isaac Yee, "Tens of Thousands of Singapore's Migrant Workers Are Infected. The Rest Are Stuck in Their Dorms as the Country Opens Up," CNN, May 14, 2020; https://www.cnn.com/2020/05/14/asia/singapore-migrant-worker-coronavirus-intl-hnk/index.html.

105   Natasha Turak, "The Gulf's Migrant Workers Are Being Exploited amid the Coronavirus Crisis, Rights Groups Say," CNBC, July 14, 2020; https://www.cnbc.com/2020/07/14/coronavirus-and-human-rights-gulfs-migrant-workers-exploited-amid-pandemic.html; Delphine Strauss, "Tens of Millions of Migrant Workers Face Job Losses and Poverty," *Financial Times*, June 24, 2020; https://app.ft.com/content/c01a38f4-f314-4232-afcc-bdbb7aa0b130

106   Soutik Biswas, "India Coronavirus: How Kerala's Covid 'Success Story' Came Undone," BBC, July 20, 2020; https://www.bbc.com/news/world-asia-india-53431672.

107   Maya Averbuch, "With Coronavirus Spreading, Mexico Vowed to Empty Detention Centers—But Migrants Were Thrust Into Chaos and Danger," *The Intercept*, May 11, 2020; https://theintercept.com/2020/05/11/coronavirus-migrants-mexico/.

108   Silvia Foster-Frau, "First Coronavirus Cases in a 'Remain in Mexico' Migrant Camp," *San Antonio Express-News*, June 30, 2020; https://www.expressnews.com/news/us-world/border-mexico/article/First-coronavirus-case-in-a-Remain-in-15376600.php.

109   "The Dark History of 'Gasoline Baths' at the Border," Vox, YouTube, July 29, 2019; https://www.youtube.com/watch?v=tkD6QfeRil8.

110   Efi Koutsokosta, "Greece Faces Fresh Calls to Probe Migrant Deaths at Its Turkish Border," *Euronews*, July 7, 2020; https://www.euronews.com/2020/07/07/greece-faces-fresh-calls-to-probe-migrant-deaths-at-its-turkish-border.

111   Transnational Institute, *COVID-19 and Border Politics*, July 2020; https://www.tni.org/files/publication-downloads/tni-covid-19-and-border-politics-brief.pdf.

112   Amnesty International, "Libya: Renewal of Migration Deal Confirms Italy's Complicity in Torture of Migrants and Refugees," January 30, 2020; https://www.amnesty.org/en/latest/news/2020/01/libya-renewal-of-migration-deal-confirms-italys-complicity-in-torture-of-migrants-and-refugees/; Sertan Sanderson, "Pope Francis Compares Libyan Camps to Concentration Camps," InfoMigrants, July 9, 2020; https://www.infomigrants.net/en/post/25920/pope-francis-compares-libyan-camps-to-concentration-camps.

113 Todd Miller, *More Than a Wall*, Transnational Institute, September 16, 2019; https://www.tni.org/en/morethanawall.

114 World Bank, "Groundswell: Preparing for Internal Climate Migration," March 19, 2018; https://www.worldbank.org/en/news/infographic/2018/03/19/groundswell---preparing-for-internal-climate-migration.

115 Abrahm Lustgarten, "The Great Climate Migration," *The New York Times*, July 23, 2020; https://www.nytimes.com/interactive/2020/07/23/magazine/climate-migration.html.

116 Miranda Cady Hallett, "How Climate Change Is Driving Emigration from Central America," PBS, September 8, 2019; https://www.pbs.org/newshour/world/how-climate-change-is-driving-emigration-from-central-america.

117 Environmental Justice Foundation, *Climate Displacement in Bangladesh*, https://ejfoundation.org/reports/climate-displacement-in-bangladesh.

118 Marta Rodriguez Martinez and Lillo Montalto Monella, "Extreme Weather Exiles: How Climate Change Is Turning Europeans into Migrants," *Euronews*, June 17, 2020; https://www.euronews.com/2020/02/26/extreme-weather-exiles-how-climate-change-is-turning-europeans-into-migrants.

119 International Labour Organization, "Labour Migration," https://www.ilo.org/global/topics/labour-migration/lang--en/index.htm.

120 Robin Millard, "Millions of Migrant Workers Head Home Due to Virus: UN," *The Jakarta Post*, June 25, 2020; https://www.thejakartapost.com/news/2020/06/25/millions-of-migrant-workers-head-home-due-to-virus-un.html.

121 Lauren Leatherby, "How the U.S. Compares With the World's Worst Coronavirus Hot Spots," *The New York Times*, July 24, 2020; https://www.nytimes.com/interactive/2020/07/23/us/coronavirus-hotspots-countries.html.

122 Shikha Silliman Bhattacharjee, *Advancing Gender Justice on Asian Fast Fashion Supply Chains Post COVID-19*, Global Labor Justice, 2020; https://globallaborjustice.org/advancing-gender-justice-on-asian-fast-fashion-supply-chains-post-covid-19/.

123 Annie Chapman, "A Doctor's Story: Inside the 'Living Hell' of Moria Refugee Camp," *The Guardian*, February 9, 2020; https://www.theguardian.com/world/2020/feb/09/moria-refugee-camp-doctors-story-lesbos-greece.

124 WatchTheMed Alarm Phone, "The Struggle of Migrant Women across the Mediterranean Sea," *American Quarterly*, Vol. 71, No. 4 (December 2019).

125 "Thousands of Black Lives Matter Protesters in Britain Demand Justice for Drowned Somali Refugee," *The National*, June 28, 2020; https://www.thenational.ae/world/europe/thousands-of-black-lives-matter-protesters-in-britain-demand-justice-for-drowned-somali-refugee-1.1040224.

126 Astrid Galvan, "For Immigrants, Marching with Black Lives Matter Has Risks," PBS, June 16, 2020; https://www.pbs.org/newshour/nation/for-immigrants-marching-with-black-lives-matter-has-risks.

127 John Burnett, "Border Patrol Response To Portland Unrest: Straying From Mission Or Continuing One?" NPR, July 23, 2020; https://www.npr.org/2020/07/23/894712004/border-patrol-response-to-portland-unrest-straying-from-mission-or-continuing-on; Todd Miller, "Border Agents Are Allowed to Operate 100 miles inside the US. That Should Worry Us," *The Guardian*, August 8, 2020; https://www.theguardian.com/commentisfree/2020/aug/08/border-agents-us-force.

128 National Priorities Project, "Trade-Offs: Your Money, Your Choices," https://www.nationalpriorities.org/interactive-data/trade-offs/?state=00&program=46.

129 Aaron Mehta, "Global Defense Spending Sees Biggest Spike in a Decade," *Defense-News*, April 27, 2020; https://www.defensenews.com/global/2020/04/27/global-defense-spending-sees-biggest-spike-in-a-decade/.

130 Lawrence Korb, "The Pentagon's Fiscal Year 2021 Budget More Than Meets U.S. National Security Needs," Center for American Priorities, May 6, 2020; https://www.americanprogress.org/issues/security/reports/2020/05/06/484620/pentagons-fiscal-year-2021-budget-meets-u-s-national-security-needs/.

131 "France FY Defense Budget, 2020—Analysis, Key Trends & Challenges," *Business Wire*, March 5, 2020; https://www.businesswire.com/news/home/20200305005640/en/France-FY-Defense-Budget-2020---Analysis.

132 Maciej Szopa, "Poland Increases Defence Expenditure By Over 11% in 2020," Defence24, January 20, 2020; https://www.defence24.com/poland-2020-defence-expenditure-almost-pln-50-billion.

133 "2021 Defence Spending to Reach 1.66 pc of GDP in Hungary," *Daily News Hungary*, July 6, 2020; https://dailynewshungary.com/2021-defence-spending-to-reach-1-66-pc-of-gdp-in-hungary/.

134 Bonnie Glaser, Matthew Funaiole, and Brian Hart, "Breaking Down China's 2020 Defense Budget," CSIS, May 22, 2020; https://www.csis.org/analysis/breaking-down-chinas-2020-defense-budget.

135 Amna Javed, "How India Hoodwinks the World about Its Real Military Budget," *Modern Diplomacy*, May 8, 2020; https://moderndiplomacy.eu/2020/05/08/how-india-hoodwinks-the-world-about-its-real-military-budget/; Sher Bano, "Pakistan's Military Spending and Defence Budget 2020-21," *Modern Diplomacy*, July 14, 2020; https://moderndiplomacy.eu/2020/07/14/pakistans-military-spending-and-defence-budget-2020-21/; Natalia Scalzaretto, "Brazil's 2021 Budget: Can the Belt Get Any Tighter?" *The Brazilian Report*, August 19, 2020; https://brazilian.report/power/2020/08/19/brazil-2021-budget-can-belt-get-any-tighter/.

136 "Россия увеличила расходы на оборону до нового рекорда," Finanz.ru, July 14, 2020; https://www.finanz.ru/novosti/aktsii/rossiya-uvelichila-raskhody-na-oboronu-do-novogo-rekorda-1029393592; Gabrielle Tétrault-Farber and Darya Korsunskaya, "Russia, Hit by Coronavirus Crisis, Considers Military Spending Cuts," Reuters, July 21, 2020; https://www.usnews.com/news/world/articles/2020-07-21/russia-hit-by-coronavirus-crisis-considers-military-spending-cuts.

137 Jr Ng, "South Korea Cuts 2020 Defence Budget to Address Covid-19," *Asian Military Review*, April 28, 2020; https://asianmilitaryreview.com/2020/04/south-korea-cuts-2020-defence-budget-to-address-covid-19/.

138 Jeff Abramson, "U.S. Fuels Growing Arms Market," *Arms Control Today*, April 2020; https://www.armscontrol.org/act/2020-04/news/us-fuels-growing-arms-market; Aaron Mehta, "To Keep Weapon Sales in Place, US Offers New Options for Payment," *Defense News*, August 4, 2020; https://www.defensenews.com/pentagon/2020/08/04/to-keep-weapon-sales-in-place-us-offers-new-options-for-payment/.

139 Nikko Dizon, "Duterte and His Generals: A Shock and Awe Response to the Pandemic," *Rappler*, July 31, 2020; https://rappler.com/newsbreak/in-depth/duterte-shock-and-awe-coronavirus-pandemic-response-generals.

140 Paige Williams, "Urgent Care from the Army Corps of Engineers," *The New Yorker*, July 27, 2020; https://www.newyorker.com/magazine/2020/08/03/urgent-care-from-the-army-corps-of-engineers; Harry Lye, "The Defence Industry's Response to Covid-19," Global Defence Technology; June 20, 2020; https://defence.nridigital.com/global_defence_technology_jun20/defence-industry-covid19-response.

141 Robert Schlesinger, "The Origins of That Eisenhower 'Every Gun That Is Made . . .' Quote," *U.S. News and World Report*, September 30, 2011; https://www.usnews.com/opinion/blogs/robert-schlesinger/2011/09/30/the-origins-of-that-eisenhower-every-gun-that-is-made-quote.

142 Carla Babb, "USS Theodore Roosevelt Deploys to Philippine Sea After COVID-19 Outbreak," VOA, May 21, 2020; https://www.voanews.com/covid-19-pandemic/uss-theodore-roosevelt-deploys-philippine-sea-after-covid-19-outbreak.

143 John Feffer, "Okinawa: Will the Pandemic Transform U.S. Military Bases?" *Responsible Statecraft*, July 17, 2020; https://responsiblestatecraft.org/2020/07/17/okinawa-will-the-pandemic-transform-u-s-military-bases/.

144 Michael Klare, "A World of 'Killer Robots' But Not 'National Security,'" *TomDispatch*, July 19, 2020; https://www.tomdispatch.com/blog/176729/tomgram%3A_michael_klare%2C_a_world_of_%22killer_robots%22_but_not_%22national_security%22.

145 David Barno and Nora Bensahel, "Five Ways the U.S. Military Will Change After the Pandemic," *War on the Rocks*, April 28, 2020; https://warontherocks.com/2020/04/five-ways-the-u-s-military-will-change-after-the-pandemic/.

146 Brad Lendon, "US Air Force pulls bombers from Guam," CNN, April 25, 2020; https://edition.cnn.com/2020/04/24/asia/guam-us-air-force-bombers-pull-out-intl-hnk/index.html.

147 Missy Ryan, Karen DeYoung, and Loveday Morris, "Pentagon Plan Will Move Troops from Germany to Italy, Belgium and Back to U.S.," *The Washington Post*, July 29, 2020; https://www.washingtonpost.com/national-security/us-troop-withdrawal-germany/2020/07/29/f5d23982-d19f-11ea-af07-1d058ca137ae_story.html.

148 Nikos Chysoloras, "Germany, France Push for Tighter EU Defense Amid U.S. Strain," *Bloomberg Quint*, June 15, 2020; https://www.bloombergquint.com/politics/germany-france-push-for-tighter-eu-defense-amid-u-s-tension; Jeroen Dobber, "EU Budget 2021-2027: What's in It for Europe's Defence?" Friedrich Naumann Stiftung, August 3, 2020; https://www.freiheit.org/security-and-defence-policy-eu-budget-2021-2027-whats-it-europes-defence.

149 "Spain Approves €7.3 Billion in Defense Spending Programs," *The Defense Post*, December 14, 2018; https://www.thedefensepost.com/2018/12/14/spain-defense-spending-7-billion/.

150 Robert Pollin and Heidi Garrett-Peltier, "The U.S. Employment Effects of Military and Domestic Spending Priorities: 2011 Update," PERI, November 28, 2011; https://www.peri.umass.edu/publication/item/449-the-u-s-employment-effects-of-military-and-domestic-spending-priorities-2011-update; Heidi Peltier, "Cut Military Spending, Fund Green Manufacturing," Watson Institute, November 13, 2019; https://watson.brown.edu/costsofwar/files/cow/imce/papers/2019/Peltier%20Nov2019%20Short%20GND%20CoW.pdf.

151 Ava Patricia Avila, "Philippine Defense Spending 2019: What's in the Data?" *Rappler*, May 28, 2020; https://www.adas.ph/2020/05/28/analysis-philippine-defense-

spending-2019-whats-in-the-data/; Research and Markets, "Philippines Defense Market Study, 2019-2024—Defense Expenditure Anticipated to Register a CAGR of 8.98%, Reaching $5.3 Billion in 2024," January 31, 2020; https://www.globenewswire.com/news-release/2020/01/31/1978090/0/en/Philippines-Defense-Market-Study-2019-2024-Defense-Expenditure-Anticipated-to-Register-a-CAGR-of-8-98-Reaching-5-3-Billion-in-2024.html.

152 Kimberly Amadeo, "2009 GDP Statistics, Growth, and Updates by Quarter," *The Balance*, April 8, 2020; https://www.thebalance.com/2009-gdp-statistics-3306037.

153 "U.S. Military Spending from 2000 to 2019," *Statista*; https://www.statista.com/statistics/272473/us-military-spending-from-2000-to-2012/.

154 The Conference Board, "The Conference Board Economic Forecast for the US Economy—August 2020," August 13, 2020; https://conference-board.org/research/us-forecast.

155 Magda Majkowska-Tomkin, "Countries Are Suspending Immigration Detention Due to Coronavirus. Let's Keep It that Way," *Euronews*, April 29, 2020; https://www.euronews.com/2020/04/29/countries-suspending-immigration-detention-due-to-coronavirus-let-s-keep-it-that-way-view.

156 Colin Woodard, "The Coolest Shipyard in America," *Politico*, July 21, 2016; https://www.politico.com/magazine/story/2016/07/philadelphia-what-works-navy-yard-214072.

157 Drew Harwell, "Google to Drop Pentagon AI Contract after Employee Objections to the 'Business of War,'" *The Washington Post*, June 1, 2018; https://www.washingtonpost.com/news/the-switch/wp/2018/06/01/google-to-drop-pentagon-ai-contract-after-employees-called-it-the-business-of-war/.

158 Andrew Smith, "Time for a Just Transition," CAAT Blog, May 21, 2020; https://blog.caat.org.uk/2020/05/21/time-for-a-just-transition/.

159 Campaign Against Arms Trade, *Arms to Renewables*, October 2014; https://www.caat.org.uk/campaigns/arms-to-renewables/arms-to-renewables-background-briefing.pdf.

160 Robinson Meyer, "Voters Really Care about Climate Change," *The Atlantic*, February 21, 2020; https://www.theatlantic.com/science/archive/2020/02/poll-us-voters-really-do-care-about-climate-change/606907/; Kathy Frankovic, "Americans Disapprove of US Withdrawing from the World Health Organization," YouGov, June 3, 2020; https://today.yougov.com/topics/politics/articles-reports/2020/06/03/americans-disapprove-us-withdrawing-world-health-0.

161 William Hartung, "What Make Us Safer," *TomDispatch*, July 7, 2020; https://www.tomdispatch.com/blog/176723/tomgram%3A_william_hartung%2C_what_makes_us_safer.

162 Ben Ndugga-Kabuye and Rachel Gilmer, "A Vision for Black Lives," Movement for Black Lives; https://m4bl.org/wp-content/uploads/2020/05/CutMilitaryExpendituresOnePager.pdf; National Priorities Project, "The Militarized Budget 2020," June 22, 2020; https://www.nationalpriorities.org/analysis/2020/militarized-budget-2020/; Brian Barrett, "The Pentagon's Hand-Me-Downs Helped Militarize Police. Here's How," *Wired*, June 2, 2020; https://www.wired.com/story/pentagon-hand-me-downs-militarize-police-1033-program/.

163 Joe Gould, "Defund Pentagon Effort Holds Message for Biden," *DefenseNews*, July 20, 2020; https://www.defensenews.com/congress/2020/07/20/defund-pentagon-ef-

fort-holds-message-for-biden/.

164 Joe Gould, "Progressive Effort to Cut Defense Fails Twice in Congress," *Defense-News*, July 22, 2020; https://www.defensenews.com/congress/2020/07/22/progressive-effort-to-cut-defense-fails-twice-in-congress/.

165 Hanna Ziady, "BP Will Slash Oil Production by 40% and Pour Billions into Green Energy," CNN, August 4, 2020; https://www.cnn.com/2020/08/04/business/bp-oil-clean-energy/index.html.

166 Tamara Lorincz, "Demilitarization for Deep Decarbonization," International Peace Bureau, September 2014; http://www.ipb.org/wp-content/uploads/2017/03/Green_Booklet_working_paper_17.09.2014.pdf.

167 Global Campaign on Military Spending, "GDAMS Healthcare Not Warfare Infographic," May 2020; https://demilitarize.org/resources/gdams-healthcare-not-warfare-infographic/.

168 Humanitarian Disarmament, "Open Letter on COVID-19 and Humanitarian Disarmament," June 2020; https://humanitariandisarmament.org/covid-19-2/open-letter-on-covid-and-humanitarian-disarmament/.

169 United Nations Secretary-General, "Secretary-General's Appeal for Global Ceasefire," March 23, 2020; https://www.un.org/sg/en/content/sg/statement/2020-03-23/secretary-generals-appeal-for-global-ceasefire.

170 Govinda Clayton, "The U.N. Has Appealed for a Global Coronavirus Cease-Fire," *The Washington Post*, April 13, 2020; https://www.washingtonpost.com/politics/2020/04/13/un-has-appealed-global-coronavirus-ceasefire/; International Crisis Group, "Global Ceasefire Call Deserves UN Security Council's Full Support," April 9, 2020; https://www.crisisgroup.org/global/global-ceasefire-call-deserves-un-security-councils-full-support.

171 Relief Web, "Statement of Support by 171 UN Member States, Non-Member Observer States, and Observers to the UN Secretary-General's Appeal for a Global Ceasefire amid the COVID-19 Pandemic," June 24, 2020; https://reliefweb.int/report/world/statement-support-171-un-member-states-non-member-observer-states-and-observers-un.

172 Kylie Atwood, "US Blocks UN Resolution on Global Coronavirus Ceasefire after China Pushes WHO Mention," CNN, May 9, 2020; https://www.cnn.com/2020/05/09/politics/us-rejects-un-coronavirus-resolution-china-who/index.html; Amnesty International, "UN Security Council Calls for a Global Ceasefire to Tackle COVID-19," July 1, 2020; https://www.amnesty.org/en/latest/news/2020/07/un-security-council-calls-for-a-global-ceasefire-to-tackle-covid-19/.

173 Caleb Quinley, "In Thailand's Deep South Conflict, a 'Glimpse of Hope', but No Momentum to Sustain a COVID-19 Ceasefire," *The New Humanitarian*, August 3, 2020; https://www.thenewhumanitarian.org/news/2020/08/03/Thailand-deep-south-conflict-coronavirus-ceasefire.

174 Ngala Killian Chimtom, "Cameroon's Deadly Mix of War and Coronavirus," BBC, May 10, 2020; https://www.bbc.com/news/world-africa-52551848n; Richard Sisk, "Opposing Russian and Syrian Mercenary Armies Face Off in Libya's Civil War," Military.com, July 19, 2020; https://www.military.com/daily-news/2020/07/19/opposing-russian-and-syrian-mercenary-armies-face-off-libyas-civil-war.html.

175 ACLED, "Call Unanswered: A Review of Responses to the UN Appeal for a Global Ceasefire," May 13, 2020, https://reliefweb.int/sites/reliefweb.int/files/resources/

acleddata.com-Call%20Unanswered%20A%20Review%20of%20Responses%20
to%20the%20UN%20Appeal%20for%20a%20Global%20Ceasefire.pdf.

176   Oxfam International, "Efforts to Forge a Global Ceasefire a 'Catastrophic
       Failure,' Says Oxfam," May 12, 2020; https://www.oxfam.
       org/en/press-releases/ef-
       forts-forge-global-ceasefire-catastrophic-failure-says-oxfam.

177   John O'Loughlin and Cullen Hendrix, "Will Climate Change Lead to More World
       Conflict?" *The Washington Post*, July 11, 2020; https://www.washingtonpost.com/
       politics/2019/07/11/how-does-climate-change-impact-conflict-world/.

178   Stephen Snyder, "Why Broken Ceasefires Are Actually Good for Peace," PRI,
       October 24, 2016; https://www.pri.org/stories/2016-10-20/why-broken-ceasefires-
       are-not-all-bad.

179   Kroc Institute for International Peace Studies, "Peace Accords Matrix," July 29, 2015;
       https://peaceaccords.nd.edu/research.

180   UN Women, "Facts and Figures: Peace and Security," https://www.unwomen.org/
       en/what-we-do/peace-and-security/facts-and-figures#_Notes.

181   Carlotta Gall, "Erdogan and Trump Form New Bond as Interests Align," *The New
       York Times*, June 10, 2020; https://www.nytimes.com/2020/06/10/world/europe/
       erdogan-trump-turkey-libya-syria.html; "Yemen war: Trump Vetoes Bill to End US
       Support for Saudi-Led Coalition," BBC, April 17, 2019; https://www.bbc.com/news/
       world-us-canada-47958014.

182   Omar Suleiman, "America's Problem With Policing Doesn't Stop at the U.S. Bor-
       der," *The Intercept*, July 21, 2020; https://theintercept.com/2020/07/21/accountabili-
       ty-drones-military-overseas-civilians/.

183   Zach Dorfman, Kim Zetter, Jenna McLaughlin, and Sean D. Naylor, "Exclusive:
       Secret Trump Order Gives CIA More Powers to Launch Cyberattacks," *Yahoo
       News*, July 15, 2020; https://news.yahoo.com/secret-trump-order-gives-cia-more-
       powers-to-launch-cyberattacks-090015219.html.

184   Alex Ward, "Mysterious Explosions Keep Happening in Iran. Israel Is Likely Be-
       hind It," *Vox*, July, 17 2020; https://www.vox.com/2020/7/17/21325985/iran-israel-ex-
       plosion-natanz-nuclear-missile.

185   John Feffer, "The Widening Rift Between the US and China," *The Nation*, April 8,
       2019; https://www.thenation.com/article/archive/china-us-xi-jinping-congagement/.

186   U.S. State Department, "Joint Declaration between the Islamic Republic of Afghan-
       istan and the United States of America for Bringing Peace to Afghanistan," Febru-
       ary 29, 2020; https://www.state.gov/wp-content/uploads/2020/02/02.29.20-US-Af-
       ghanistan-Joint-Declaration.pdf.

187   Ahmad Mukhtar, "Afghanistan Frees Dozens More 'Dangerous' Taliban Prisoners
       in the Name of Peace," CBS News, August 14, 2020; https://www.cbsnews.com/
       news/afghanistan-frees-dozens-more-dangerous-taliban-prisoners-in-the-name-of-
       peace/.

188   Susannah George and Aziz Tassal, "As Afghanistan Struggles to Start Peace
       Talks, Violence Fills the Void," *The Washington Post*, August 10, 2020; https://www.
       washingtonpost.com/world/asia_pacific/spike-in-violence-fills-void-in-afghanistan-
       during-peace-talks-delay/2020/08/09/97a251fc-d3fd-11ea-826b-cc394d824e35_story.
       html.

189   Andrew Quilty, "Afghanistan's Unseen Covid Crisis," *The Interpreter*, August
       12, 2020; https://www.lowyinstitute.org/the-interpreter/afghanistan-s-un-

seen-covid-crisis.

190 Gabriela Bernal, "North Korea Steps up Its War on COVID-19," *The Diplomat*, August 6, 2020; https://thediplomat.com/2020/08/north-korea-steps-up-its-war-on-covid-19/.

191 Mike Yeo, "Japan Suspends Aegis Ashore Deployment, Pointing to Cost and Technical Issues," *DefenseNews*, June 15, 2020; https://www.defensenews.com/global/asia-pacific/2020/06/15/japan-suspends-aegis-ashore-deployment-pointing-to-cost-and-technical-issues/.

192 "Jared Kushner Insists Middle East Peace Plan Is 'a Real Effort to Break Logjam,'" *The Guardian*, February 2, 2020; https://www.theguardian.com/us-news/2020/feb/02/jared-kushner-middle-east-peace-plan.

193 Danny Zaken, "Israel, UAE Test Potential for Cooperation on COVID-19," *Al-Monitor*, July 9, 2020; https://www.al-monitor.com/pulse/originals/2020/07/israel-united-arab-emirates-palestinians-benjamin-netanyahu.html#ixzz6WeoRpsqb.

194 Peter Beaumont, "Death Toll in Yemen war Reaches 100,000," *The Guardian*, October 31, 2019; https://www.theguardian.com/world/2019/oct/31/death-toll-in-yemen-war-reaches-100000.

195 Mercy Corps, "The Facts: What You Need to Know about the Crisis in Yemen," July 17, 2020; https://reliefweb.int/report/yemen/facts-what-you-need-know-about-crisis-yemen; "IOM: Over 100,000 Yemenis Have Been Displaced Since Beginning of 2020," *Middle East Monitor*, July 22, 2020; https://www.middleeastmonitor.com/20200722-iom-over-100000-yemenis-have-been-displaced-since-beginning-of-2020/.

196 Omer Karasapan, "Yemen and COVID-19: The Pandemic Exacts Its Devastating Toll," Brookings, June 15, 2020; https://www.brookings.edu/blog/future-development/2020/06/15/yemen-and-covid-19-the-pandemic-exacts-its-devastating-toll/.

197 Sam Kiley, "Yemen Coronavirus: Experts Fear Nation Could Suffer One of the World's Worst Outbreaks," CNN, June 5, 2020; https://www.msn.com/en-us/news/world/yemen-coronavirus-experts-fear-nation-could-suffer-one-of-the-worlds-worst-outbreaks/ar-BB152Reo.

198 Ethan Azad, "Now Is Not the Time to Withhold Aid to Yemen," *Responsible Statecraft*, August 4, 2020; https://responsiblestatecraft.org/2020/08/04/now-is-not-the-time-to-withhold-aid-to-yemen/.

199 Paul Holtom et al., *United Nations Arms Embargoes Their Impact on Arms Flows and Target Behaviour*, SIPRI, January 2007; https://www.researchgate.net/publication/265643465_UNITED_NATIONS_ARMS_EMBARGOES_THEIR_IMPACT_ON_ARMS_FLOWS_AND_TARGET_BEHAVIOUR.

200 Charles Tiefer, "State IG Did Not Clear Pompeo About The Wrongful Arms Sales To Saudi Arabia," *Forbes*, August 10, 2020; https://www.forbes.com/sites/charlestiefer/2020/08/10/state-ig-did-not-clear-pompeo-about-the-wrongful-arms-sales-to-saudi-arabis/#1d69d02a6fd3.

201 United Nations Peacekeeping, "Where We Operate," https://peacekeeping.un.org/en/where-we-operate.

202 United Nations Peacekeeping, "Historical Timeline of UN Peacekeeping," https://peacekeeping.un.org/en/historical-timeline-of-un-peacekeeping.

203 Carol Morello, "Trump Shrugs as U.N. Warns It's about to Run Out of Money," *The*

Washington Post, October 9, 2019; https://www.washingtonpost.com/national-security/trump-shrugs-as-un-warns-its-about-to-run-out-of-money/2019/10/09/568f8756-eac5-11e9-85c0-85a098e47b37_story.html.

204 Zoe McAlister, "'Doctors Without Borders' Sent Team to Help Navajo Nation," *Newswire*, May 14, 2020; https://newswire.net/newsroom/news/00119567-first-time-in-the-us-doctors-without-borders-visited-navajo-indians.html.

205 Peace Direct, "COVID-19 and Local Peacebuilding," April 8, 2020; https://www.peacedirect.org/us/publications/covid19andpeacebuilding/.

206 Alex Ward, "Anti-Lockdown Protests Aren't Just an American Thing. They're a Global Phenomenon," *Vox*, May 20, 2020; https://www.vox.com/2020/5/20/21263919/anti-lockdown-protests-coronavirus-germany-brazil-uk-chile; Alexander Marrow and Maria Tsvetkova, "Hundreds Protest in Southern Russian against Coronavirus Curbs," Reuters, April 20, 2020; https://www.reuters.com/article/us-health-coronavirus-russia-protests/hundreds-protest-in-southern-russian-against-coronavirus-curbs-idUSKBN22225B.

207 Oren Liebermann, Milena Veselinovic, and Emma Reynolds, "Huge Protests Rock Several Countries as Coronavirus Ignites Rage against Governments," CNN, July 15, 2020; https://www.cnn.com/2020/07/15/world/protests-israel-serbia-bulgaria-coronavirus-intl/index.html; John Feffer, "COVID-19 and the End of Autocrats," Foreign Policy In Focus, August 26, 2020; https://fpif.org/covid-19-and-the-end-of-autocrats/; Enrico Dela Cruz, "Philippine Protesters Rally over Controversial Anti-Terror Bill," Reuters, June 12, 2020; https://www.reuters.com/article/us-philippines-rights-protests/philippine-protesters-rally-over-controversial-anti-terror-bill-idUSKBN23J1FG.

208 Robin Wright, "The Story of 2019: Protests in Every Corner of the Globe," *The New Yorker*, December 30, 2019; https://www.newyorker.com/news/our-columnists/the-story-of-2019-protests-in-every-corner-of-the-globe.

209 Gregory Warner, "So Long, Black Pete," NPR, June 24, 2020; https://www.npr.org/2020/06/24/882816031/so-long-black-pete; Lauren Frayer, "India Sees A Change Sparked By Black Lives Matter Movement," NPR, June 29, 2020; https://www.npr.org/2020/06/29/884958682/india-sees-a-change-sparked-by-black-lives-matter-movement.

210 Yelena Dzhanova, "Protests against Police Brutality Pop Up in Small Towns in Trump-Friendly Regions," CNBC, June 8, 2020; https://www.cnbc.com/2020/06/08/police-brutality-protests-pop-up-in-small-towns-in-trump-country.html.

211 John Campbell, "Black Lives Matter Protests in Africa Shine a Light on Local Police Brutality," Council on Foreign Relations, July 8, 2020; https://www.cfr.org/blog/black-lives-matter-protests-africa-shine-light-local-police-brutality.

212 Eduardo Campos Lima, "Black Lives Matter Is Inspiring Demonstrations all over Latin America," *America Magazine*, June 22, 2020; https://www.americamagazine.org/politics-society/2020/06/22/black-lives-matter-movement-latin-america-protests.

213 "Southeast Asia on the Black Lives Matter Protests: How They Covered It," *ASEAN Today*, June 6, 2020; https://www.aseantoday.com/2020/06/southeast-asia-on-the-black-lives-matter-protests-how-they-covered-it/.

214 Jason Burke, "Burundi President Dies of Illness Suspected To Be Coronavirus," *The*

Guardian, June 9, 2020; https://www.theguardian.com/world/2020/jun/09/burundi-president-dies-illness-suspected-coronavirus-pierre-nkurunziz.

215 Rod Austin, "'If We Don't Kill These People, They Will Kill You': Policing Africa's Largest Slum," *The Guardian*, August 6, 2019; https://www.theguardian.com/global-development/2019/aug/06/if-we-dont-kill-these-people-they-will-kill-you-policing-africas-largest-slum.

216 Danielle Paquette, "Mali Coup Leader was Trained by U.S. Military," *The Washington Post*, August 21, 2020; https://www.washingtonpost.com/world/asia_pacific/mali-coup-leader-was-trained-by-us-special-operations-forces/2020/08/21/33153fbe-e31c-11ea-82d8-5e55d47e90ca_story.html.

217 ITUC-CSI, "Global Business, Workers and Civil Society Call for Comprehensive Emergency Debt Relief to Enable All Countries in Need to Combat the COVID-19 Pandemic," July 13, 2020; https://www.ituc-csi.org/covid-19-debt-relief; ITUC-CSI, "Reform the IMF and World Bank to Re-Build Better from COVID-19," May 21, 2020; https://www.ituc-csi.org/reform-imf-word-bank-covid-19.

218 Public Services International, "'We Health Workers Must Not Become Coronavirus Martyrs'—Nurse George Poe Williams," March 16, 2020; https://publicservices.international/resources/videos/we-health-workers-must-not-become-coronavirus-martyrs---nurse-george-poe-williams?id=9561&lang=en&affiliate_id=700.

219 Africans Rising, "African Feminist Post-COVID-19 Economic Recovery Statement," https://www.africans-rising.org/african-feminist-post-covid-19-economic-recovery-statement/.

220 ITUC-CSI, "A Global Social Protection Fund Is Possible," June 29, 2020; https://www.ituc-csi.org/global-social-protection-fund.

221 Olivier Balch, "Buen Vivir: the Social Philosophy Inspiring Movements in South America," *The Guardian*, February 4, 2013; https://www.theguardian.com/sustainable-business/blog/buen-vivir-philosophy-south-america-eduardo-gudynas.

222 Robert Roos, "Experts: SARS sparked global cooperation to fight disease," CIDRAP, April 13, 2015; https://www.cidrap.umn.edu/news-perspective/2013/04/experts-sars-sparked-global-cooperation-fight-disease.

223 Ibid.

224 Selam Gebrekidan, "The World Has a Plan to Fight Coronavirus. Most Countries Are Not Using It," *The New York Times*, March 12, 2020; https://www.nytimes.com/2020/03/12/world/coronavirus-world-health-organization.html.

225 Keith Bradsher, "China's Economy Rebounds From Coronavirus, but Shares Fall," *The New York Times*, July 15, 2020; https://www.nytimes.com/2020/07/15/business/economy/china-coronavirus-economy.html.

226 Amitav Acharya and Barry Buzan, *The Making of Global International Relations* (Cambridge: Cambridge University Press, 2019).

227 Rachel Brown, Heather Hurlburt, and Alexandra Stark, "How the Coronavirus Sows Civil Conflict," *Foreign Affairs*, June 6, 2020; https://www.foreignaffairs.com/articles/world/2020-06-06/how-coronavirus-sows-civil-conflict.

228 Demetri Sevastopulo and Katrina Manson, "Trump Escalates Anti-China Campaign with Hong Kong Sanctions," *Financial Times*, August 8, 2020; https://www.ft.com/content/6822dffd-8cb8-494d-9a89-c6ee29a345d4;

Ana Swanson, Mike Isaac, and Paul Mozur, "Trump Targets WeChat and TikTok, in

Sharp Escalation With China," *The New York Times*, August 6, 2020; https://www.nytimes.com/2020/08/06/technology/trump-wechat-tiktok-china.html; Pranshu Verma and Edward Wong, "U.S. Imposes Sanctions on Chinese Officials Over Mass Detention of Muslims," *The New York Times*, July 9, 2020; https://www.nytimes.com/2020/07/09/world/asia/trump-china-sanctions-uighurs.html.

229   Idrees Ali and Phil Stewart, "Pentagon Chief Expresses Concern to Chinese Counterpart about Beijing's Activity in South China Sea," Reuters, August 6, 2020; https://www.reuters.com/article/us-usa-china-military/pentagon-chief-expresses-concern-to-chinese-counterpart-about-beijings-activity-in-south-china-sea-idUSKCN2522T6; Hall Gardner, "The Great China-India Clash Everyone Saw Coming," *The National Interest*, July 28, 2020; https://nationalinterest.org/feature/great-china-india-clash-everyone-saw-coming-165752?page=0%2C1.

230   Mike Pompeo, "Communist China and the Free World's Future," U.S. State Department, July 23, 2020; https://www.state.gov/communist-china-and-the-free-worlds-future/; David Nakamura, "Once Reluctant to Hit China on Human Rights, Trump Moves to Use the Issue as a Cudgel amid Growing Tensions," *The Washington Post*, August 9, 2020; https://www.washingtonpost.com/politics/trump-china-human-rights/2020/08/08/b2d09172-d97b-11ea-930e-d88518c57dcc_story.html.

231   Ryan Pickrell, "Pentagon Chief Warns Beijing that the US Military Isn't 'Going to be Stopped by Anybody' from Operating in the South China Sea," *Business Insider*, July 21, 2020; https://www.businessinsider.com/us-wont-be-stopped-by-anybody-in-south-china-sea-2020-7.

232   Phuong Nguyen and Khanh Vu, "Vietnam Is Warning about Chinese Bombers Deployed to Disputed South China Sea islands," *Business Insider*, August 21, 2020; https://www.businessinsider.com/vietnam-warning-chinese-bombers-disputed-south-china-sea-islands-2020-8.

233   Marc Caputo, "Anti-China Sentiment Is on the Rise," Politico, May 20, 2020; https://www.politico.com/news/2020/05/20/anti-china-sentiment-coronavirus-poll-269373

234   United Nations, "Initiative on Financing for Development in the Era of COVID-19 and Beyond," May 28, 2020; https://www.un.org/en/coronavirus/financing-development; Alex Cobham, "UN FACTI Panel Envisages Major Global Reforms," Tax Justice Network, July 28, 2020; https://www.taxjustice.net/2020/07/28/un-facti-panel-envisages-major-global-reforms/.

235   Jessica Matthews, "The New Nuclear Threat," *The New York Review of Books*, August 20, 2020; https://www.nybooks.com/articles/2020/08/20/new-nuclear-threat/.

236   "Filipino Crew Member Commits Suicide On Cruise Ship," *Marine Insight*, June 12, 2020; https://www.marineinsight.com/shipping-news/filipino-crew-member-commits-suicide/.

237   ILO, "ILO Monitor: COVID-19 and the World of Work. Fifth edition," June 30, 2020; https://www.ilo.org/wcmsp5/groups/public/@dgreports/@dcomm/documents/briefingnote/wcms_749399.pdf.

238   ILO, *The Economics of Artificial Intelligence: Implications for the Future of Work*, October 17, 2018; https://www.ilo.org/global/topics/future-of-work/publications/research-papers/WCMS_647306/lang--en/index.htm.

239   ADB, *The Future of Work: Regional Perspectives*, May 2018; https://www.adb.org/publications/future-work-regional-perspectives.

240   Harriet Torry, "U.S. Economy Contracted at Record Rate Last Quarter; Jobless Claims Rise to 1.43 Million," *The Wall Street Journal*, July 30, 2020; https://www.wsj.com/articles/us-economy-gdp-report-second-quarter-coronavirus-11596061406; Elizabeth Lopatto, "In the Pandemic Economy, Tech Companies Are Raking It in," *The Verge*, July 30, 2020; https://www.theverge.com/2020/7/30/21348652/pandemic-earnings-antitrust-google-facebook-apple-amazon.

241   Heather Long, "The Recession Is Over for the Rich, But the Working Class Is Far from Recovered," *The Washington Post*, August 13, 2020; https://www.washingtonpost.com/business/2020/08/13/recession-is-over-rich-working-class-is-far-recovered/.

242   John Feffer, "The Pandemic Reveals a Europe More United than the United States," Foreign Policy In Focus, July 29, 2020; https://fpif.org/the-pandemic-reveals-a-europe-more-united-than-the-united-states/.

243   Richard Heydarian, "Strongman Duterte's COVID-19 Failings Usher in New Generation of Leaders," *Nikkei Asian Review*, July 22, 2020; https://asia.nikkei.com/Opinion/Strongman-Duterte-s-COVID-19-failings-usher-in-new-generation-of-leaders.

244   Satoko Kishimoto, Lavinia Steinfort, and Olivier Petitjean, eds., *The Future is Public*, Transnational Institute, May 12, 2020; https://www.tni.org/en/futureispublic.

245   Peter Peterson Foundation, "The United States Spends More on Defense than the Next Ten Countries Combined," May 15, 2020; https://www.pgpf.org/blog/2020/05/the-united-states-spends-more-on-defense-than-the-next-10-countries-combined; National Priorities Project, "A Unified Budget to Demilitarize America, At Home and Abroad," January 7, 2020; https://www.nationalpriorities.org/analysis/2020/unified-budget-demilitarize-america-home-and-abroad/.

246   Chiara Vercellone, "Who Were the Largest Major Arms Exporters in the Last 5 Years?" *DefenseNews*, March 9, 2020; https://www.defensenews.com/2020/03/09/who-were-the-largest-major-arms-exporters-in-the-last-5-years/.

247   Jeff Abramson and Greg Webb, "U.S. to Quit Arms Trade Treaty," *Arms Control Today*, May 2019; https://www.armscontrol.org/act/2019-05/news/us-quit-arms-trade-treaty.

248   World Vision, "Forced to Flee: Top Countries Refugees Are Coming From," June 19, 2020; https://www.worldvision.org/refugees-news-stories/forced-to-flee-top-countries-refugees-coming-from.

249   David Luban, "America the Unaccountable," *The New York Review of Books*, August 20, 2020; https://www.nybooks.com/articles/2020/08/20/icc-justice-america-unaccountable/.

250   "Arctic Sea Ice Melting Faster Than Forecast: Study," NDTV, August 18, 2020; https://www.ndtv.com/world-news/arctic-sea-ice-melting-faster-than-forecast-study-2281569.

251   Somini Sengupta and Julfikar Ali Manik, "A Quarter of Bangladesh Is Flooded. Millions Have Lost Everything," *The New York Times*, July 30, 2020; https://www.nytimes.com/2020/07/30/climate/bangladesh-floods.html.

252   Jacob Margolis, "An 'Unprecedented Number Of Large Fires' Have Fire Officials Warning Resources Are Getting Scarce," LAist, August 19, 2020; https://laist.com/latest/post/20200819/cal-fire-resources-wildfires-lightning-california.

253   Jubilee USA Network, "G20/IMF: Protect Vulnerable, Prevent Financial Crisis

as Covid-19 Spreads," https://www.jubileeusa.org/aa_covid-19_imf_2020_petition?utm_campaign=aa_g20_covid_aid_debt&utm_campaign=aa_g20_covid_aid_debt&utm_medium=email&utm_medium=email&utm_source=jubileeusa&utm_source=jubileeusa.

254   "Open letter to governments on ISDS and COVID-19," June 2020, http://s2bnetwork.org/wp-content/uploads/2020/06/OpenLetterOnISDSAndCOVID_June2020.pdf.

255   Climate Justice Alliance, "A People's Orientation to a Regenerative Economy," https://climatejusticealliance.org/regenerativeeconomy/.

About the Author

John Feffer is the director of Foreign Policy in Focus at the Institute for Policy Studies. He is the author, most recently, of *Aftershock: A Journey into Eastern Europe's Broken Dreams* and the *Splinterlands* trilogy.

About the Institute for Policy Studies

Based in Washington, DC, IPS is a progressive think tank dedicated to building a more equitable, ecologically sustainable, and peaceful society. In partnership with dynamic social movements, we turn transformative policy ideas into action.

About the Transnational Institute

Based in Amsterdam in the Netherlands, TNI is an international research and advocacy institute committed to building a just, democratic, and sustainable world. For more than forty years, TNI has served as a unique nexus between social movements, engaged scholars, and policy makers.

About Focus on the Global South

Focus on the Global South was established in 1995 to challenge neoliberalism, militarism and corporate-driven globalisation while strengthening just and equitable alternatives. With offices in Bangkok, New Delhi, and Manila, we work in solidarity with the Global South—the great majority of humanity that is marginalized and dispossessed by corporate-driven globalisation and global capitalism—believing that progressive social change and Global South solidarity are imperative if the needs and aspirations of oppressed peoples across the world are to be met.